Evaluating health promotion
Practice and methods

SECOND EDITION

Edited by

Margaret Thorogood and
Yolande Coombes

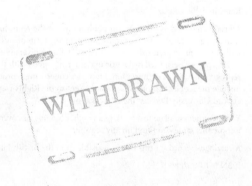
OXFORD
UNIVERSITY PRESS

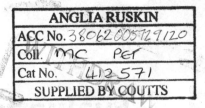
OXFORD
UNIVERSITY PRESS

Great Clarendon Street, Oxford OX2 6DP

Oxford University Press is a department of the University of Oxford.
It furthers the University's objective of excellence in research, scholarship,
and education by publishing worldwide in

Oxford New York

Auckland Cape Town Dar es Salaam Hong Kong Karachi
Kuala Lumpur Madrid Melbourne Mexico City Nairobi
New Delhi Shanghai Taipei Toronto

With offices in

Argentina Austria Brazil Chile Czech Republic France Greece
Guatemala Hungary Italy Japan South Korea Poland Portugal
Singapore Switzerland Thailand Turkey Ukraine Vietnam

Oxford is a registered trade mark of Oxford University Press
in the UK and in certain other countries

Published in the United States
by Oxford University Press Inc., New York

A catalogue record for this title is available from the British Library

ISBN 0-19-852880-9 (Pbk)

10 9 8 7 6 5 4 3

Typeset by Integra Software Services Pvt. Ltd, Pondicherry, India
Printed in Great Britain
on acid-free paper by
Ashford Colour Press Ltd, Gosport, Hampshire

Contents

Contributors

Salah Al Zaroo
Assistant Professor,
Palestine Polytechnic
University,
West Bank, Palestine

Kathryn Backett-Milburn
Professor of the Sociology of
Families and Health
Research Unit in Health,
Behaviour and Change
(RUHBC) School of Clinical
Sciences and Community
Health,
University of Edinburgh,
Teviot Place, Edinburgh

Virginia Berridge
Professor of History and
Head of Centre for History in
Public Health,
Public and Environmental
Health Research Unit,
London School of Hygiene and
Tropical Medicine

Annie Britton
Lecturer in Epidemiology,
Department of Epidemiology
and Public Health,
University College London,
and Honorary Lecturer,
Public and Environmental
Health Research Unit LSHTM

Steven Chapman
Research Director,
Population Services International,
Washington, DC

Yolande Coombes
Regional Researcher,
Population Services
International,
Nairobi, Kenya

Wendy Gnich
Research Fellow,
Research Unit in Health,
Behaviour and Change
(RUHBC) School of Clinical
Sciences and Community
Health,
University of Edinburgh

Rachel Jewkes
Chief Scientist and Director,
Gender and Health Group,
Medical Research Council,
Pretoria, South Africa

Gillian Lewando Hundt
Professor of Social Sciences
in Health,
Institute of Health, School
of Health and Social
Studies,
University of Warwick,
Coventry

Wendy Macdowall
Research Fellow,
Centre for Sexual and
Reproductive Health Research,
Public and Environmental
Health Research Unit,
London School of Hygiene and
Tropical Medicine

Dalya Marks
Lecturer,
Public and Environmental
Health Research Unit,
London School of Hygiene and
Tropical Medicine

Stephen Platt
Director,
Research Unit in Health,
Behaviour and Change
(RUHBC), School of Clinical
Sciences and Community Health,
University of Edinburgh

David Rankin
Research Fellow,
Research Unit in Health,
Behaviour and Change (RUHBC)
School of Clinical Sciences and
Community Health,
University of Edinburgh

Deborah Ritchie
Senior Lecturer,
School of Social Sciences,
Media and Communication,
Faculty of Health and Social
Sciences,
Queen Margaret University
College, Edinburgh

Warren Stevens
Health Economist,
MRC Laboratories,
Banjul, The Gambia

Margaret Thorogood
Professor of Epidemiology,
Division of Health in the
Community,
Warwick Medical School,
University of Warwick, Coventry

Julie Truman
Research Fellow,
Research Unit in Health,
Behaviour and Change
(RUHBC) School of Clinical
Sciences and Community
Health,
University of Edinburgh

Kaye Wellings
Professor of Sexual and
Reproductive Health Research,
Public and Environmental
Health Research Unit,
London School of Hygiene and
Tropical Medicine

Part I

Overview

Chapter 1

Introduction

Yolande Coombes and Margaret Thorogood

In the first edition of this book three years ago, we commented on the developments in health promotion at that time, most notably the widening boundaries of health promotion and the importance of health promotion as an emerging discipline. We stated then that health promotion 'has now reached the point where credible demonstrations of the value of its activity and its effectiveness are needed in order to sustain and expand the current position'. Since then health promotion has moved on and there has been a substantial increase in the evidence base for health promotion interventions. Further strengthening that evidence base is one of the key themes of this second edition. Three years ago we felt that unresolved theoretical and practical issues concerning the evaluation of health promotion were hampering developing the evidence base. Some of those debates have been resolved; for example, it is now accepted that both quantitative and qualitative methodologies have an important contribution to make. Others, however, persist such as interventions being evaluated using inappropriate tools. The purpose of this book remains largely unchanged. We hope that it will provide a further contribution to the evidence base while exploring a wide range of evaluation activity and highlighting the theoretical and practical problems encountered. The book offers examples of successful evaluations and suggestions for further development of this area.

Health and health promotion

There are a wide variety of concepts of health that differ between individuals, between professions, and between cultures. At one end of a spectrum health is defined as the absence of disease or longevity and at the other end health is seen as the concept of enablement or well-being. The most commonly used definition of health in health promotion is that set down by the World Health Organization: 'Health is seen as a resource for everyday life, not the object of living . . . Health is a positive concept emphasizing social and personal resources as well as physical capabilities.' (WHO 1986).

Just as health has many definitions, it is not surprising that health promotion is also defined in a number of ways. What we now understand as health promotion includes activities such as public policy aimed at improving health through legislation, regulation or policy directives; clinical interventions which aim to prevent disease (such as screening and immunization); education which aims to enable people to take informed decisions and thus take more control over their life; and a variety of interventions which aim to strengthen communities and increase social capital. All of these activities happily fit within the most commonly used definition of health promotion that was laid down in the Ottawa Charter in 1986 as 'the process of enabling people to increase control over and to improve their health' (WHO 1986). However one views health promotion and what constitutes health promotion interventions, it is clear that the past decade has seen an increase in the sophistication of the discipline and that this has brought with it the need for more rigorous evaluation and a stronger evidence base.

The evaluation of health promotion

Evaluation has become an increasingly important concept. The concepts of efficiency and cost-effectiveness are now central to the development of new initiatives in many spheres, including education and, most of all, health. Associated concepts such as quality assurance and audit have become increasingly important. The powerful evidence-based medicine movement, which insists that the randomized controlled trial is the ultimate tool for evaluation, gives more weight to the role of treatment than prevention in the debate on the relative effectiveness of the two approaches (Health Promotion International 1996). In defining itself as a new and separate discipline, health promotion has attempted to distance itself from curative medicine by focusing on an holistic approach to health (Burrows *et al.* 1995). However, in order to maintain or enhance its position as an important policy option, health promotion must engage credibly with the evidence-based medicine movement.

Evaluation means literally to place a value or to quantify the worth. The problem in evaluating health promotion is deciding how to value or quantify the outcome. One of the difficulties facing the evaluation of any health promotion activity is deciding on what value to give to 'health'. As already discussed above, the concept of health is relative and is interpreted and defined in different ways by different people. It is likely, then, that any value placed on health will be subjective and interpreted on an individual basis. It is tempting to only measure outcomes in terms that are easily quantifiable, while ignoring those outcomes that cannot be so easily quantified. The danger is that we will measure what is easily evaluable and ignore what is valuable. This is one of the challenges that faces us in developing useful and meaningful methods of evaluating health promotion and strengthening the evidence base. In this book we argue that it is not enough to simply opt out of evaluating outcomes, nor is it sufficient to concentrate on quantifiable outcome measures, such as morbidity or mortality, which are often too distal from the intervention. Most evaluations aim to demonstrate the attribution of an effect and this is most usually done by determining the exact relationship between an intervention and the outcome.

The range of activities involved in health promotion, and the multiple levels of operation, generate difficulties for its evaluation. Each type of activity demands a different form of evaluation. The issue in health promotion evaluation is the accuracy and appropriateness of measurement. This applies equally to quantitative and qualitative study designs. There cannot be just one method for the evaluation of health promotion initiatives because the initiatives themselves draw on a variety of methods and disciplines. Unfortunately, the methodologies for evaluation have sometimes been borrowed uncritically from other, more narrowly defined disciplines. As a consequence, health promotion has been evaluated using inappropriate tools, leading to unsustainable conclusions (Speller *et al.* 1997). The challenge in the next decade is to develop more accurate and appropriate measures and tools for the evaluation of a wide range of different health promotion initiatives (Mant 1996, Health Promotion International 1996, Speller 1997).

Quantitative and qualitative approaches

The unique nature of health promotion interventions requires evaluation methodologies using both qualitative and quantitative approaches. Health promotion is a particularly multidisciplinary activity – the different disciplines contributing to this book and other health promotion volumes are testament to this. It is therefore imperative that we use a range of evaluation methodologies, each suited to measuring and evaluating different interventions and activities within the overall sphere of health promotion.

Health promotion needs to establish scientific credibility if it is to enhance its position as a discipline. Using the term 'science' does not mean that quantitative methods are viewed as superior to qualitative, but that there is a need for rigour on how all methods of evaluation are used. McKinlay (1993) suggested that what we need to develop is a concept of 'appropriate methodology' for health promotion. Within this concept no one method would be rated better than another, but would be taken on their appropriateness for the job in hand; thus quantitative methods would tend to answer questions as to *whether* there is relationship and qualitative methods address *why* there is a relationship.

The importance of process evaluation

Outcome evaluation aims to determine whether there is a relationship between an activity and the outcome. But there is another, important, part of health promotion evaluation that concerns the question of why certain outcomes happen. This is the area of process evaluation. Process evaluation enables us to explore what is going on within a health promotion initiative, often producing results that are a great surprise to the researchers! Moreover, process evaluation can be used iteratively during the process of an intervention to refine and improve the methods used. Process evaluation allows the validity of the participants' viewpoint, and of the participants' value system. The Ottawa Charter viewed health promotion as a process, not an outcome – health promotion is carried out *with* people, not on them. Thus the contribution of process evaluation to strengthening the evidence base for health promotion must not be overlooked.

This book

This book argues for a broad-minded approach to developing a toolbox of methods for evaluating health promotion, using qualitative and quantitative methods, and focusing on process as well as outcome. The next chapter recounts the development of health promotion, and outlines why an historical approach to evaluation is important within the policy arena, as well as discussing the recent history of evaluation itself. Part II, Methods of evaluation, discusses some of the problems and the strengths of different methods. Chapter 3 emphasizes the need to strengthen the evidence base for health promotion and argues that this process can be done incrementally, from small-scale process evaluations through to larger outcome evaluation. It suggests that we should take a backwards approach to evaluation, starting with the question 'Why are we evaluating?' in order to guide us to the nature and scope of the evaluation that should be undertaken. Chapter 4 focuses on economic approaches to evaluation, highlighting how economic evaluation can be a powerful tool in distinguishing and proving the true value of health promotion interventions compared to disease treatment. Chapter 5 concentrates on experimental designs in health promotion evaluation. The theme of using incremental evidence is continued here and the authors suggest appropriate guidelines for when to use randomized controlled trials but highlight that such trials cannot alone provide all the evidence that we need. Chapter 6 concentrates on the role of process evaluation and its contribution to the evidence base.

Part III of the book discusses some of the isues of putting evaluation into practice. Chapter 7 focuses on the evaluation of social marketing and highlights some practical examples of evaluation of this approach; Chapter 8 concentrates on the difficulties of evaluating a sensitive and complicated topic: intimate partner violence. Chapter 9 focuses on the problems of evaluating community participation or community development initiatives. In Chapter 10 the concept of the ethics of health promotion is discussed, focusing on the issue of acquiring informed consent. Chapter 11 examines the difficulties inherent in evaluating mass media campaigns, and in particular addresses the difficulties of attribution. Finally, chapter 12 discusses the much neglected need to evaluate the process of disseminating the findings of health promotion research.

Key points

◆ Health is a subjective concept.

◆ It is difficult to evaluate health promotion activities because it is difficult measure health.

◆ Health promotion involves a variety of multi-disciplinary activities; therefore a range of methods for evaluation must be used.

◆ Rigorous evaluation methods are needed in order to strengthen the evidence base for the further development of health promotion.

References

Burrows, R., Bunton, R., Muncer, S., and Gillen, K. (1995) The efficacy of health promotion, health economics and later modernism. *Health Education Research*, **10**, 242–249.

Health Promotion International (1996). Where next for evaluation? *Health Promotion International* **11**, 171–173.

Kemm, J. and Close, A. (1995) *Health Promotion. Theory and Practice*. Macmillan, London.

Mant, D. (1996) Health promotion and disease prevention: the evaluation of health service interventions. In M. Peckham and R. Smith (eds) *Scientific Basis of Health Services*, pp. 170–178. BMJ Publishing Group, London.

McKinlay, J. B. (1993) The promotion of health through planned socio-political change: challenges for research and policy. *Social Science and Medicine*, **36** (2), 109–117.

Nutbeam, D. (1998) Evaluating health promotion – progress, problems and solutions. *Health Promotion International*, **13**, 27–44.

Seedhouse, D. (1986) *Health: Foundations for Achievement.* John Wiley and Sons.

Speller, V., Learmouth, A., and Harrison, D. (1997) The search for evidence of effective health promotion. *British Medical Journal*, **315**, 361–362.

WHO (1984) *Health Promotion: A Discussion Document on the Concept and Principles.* Copenhagen, WHO Regional Office for Europe.

WHO (1986) *Ottawa Charter for Health Promotion.* World Health Organization and Health and Welfare. Ontario, Canada.

Chapter 2

Historical and policy approaches

Virginia Berridge

Using historical approaches to evaluate 'health promotion' might just mean a history of the last twenty or so years. We could start with the 1974 Lalonde Report in Canada, *A New Perspective on the Health of Canadians*, and trace a subsequent cascade of 'milestones' in health promotion history such as the 1976 policy document, *Prevention and Health: Everybody's Business*, followed by the 1978 declaration of Alma Ata, *Health for All* from WHO in 1981 and its 38 targets for health in the European Region in 1985. The Ottawa Charter for Health Promotion followed in 1986. The Healthy Cities project was launched in 1987. In 1992 came the publication of the *Health of the Nation*, while the new British Labour government in 1997 for the first time specifically appointed a minister responsible for what it now termed 'public health'. Further initiatives have followed.

Such parades of dates and policy documents provide a sense of excitement and movement. They encourage us to think that these years have been ones of incessant activity – that progress has been made and new definitions and concepts have been established. Health promotion, as other chapters in this volume demonstrate, is essentially a fuzzy concept – but, for the purposes of this chapter, it is taken to mean the developments since the 1980s whereby the issue of individual health in relation to the environment has made its way in various forms onto the policy agenda. There is a danger that the parade of dates fronting this chapter encourages a type of 'Whig history' where all events are seen as leading to a time of greater understanding and action in the present. At a broader level, these events do little to deepen historical understanding. They do not tell much about *why* or *how* these policies have developed. This chapter will develop a historical understanding of 'health promotion' at three different levels. First, it will look at how what we now term 'health promotion' fits into changing definitions of public health and the rationales for those definitions since the eighteenth century. Then it will examine a more short-term form of historical evaluation, looking at how the 'contemporary history' of recent health promotion policies can also provide a form of evaluation. History is a questioning discipline – and so, finally, this chapter will ask, why are we talking about evaluation at all? What is the history of the concept of evaluation and why has it now come centre stage as far as health is concerned?

The long view: changing definitions of public health since the eighteenth century

Nineteenth century environmentalism

A health promotion glossary commissioned by WHO Europe defined the 'new public health' of the late twentieth century in the following terms:

> Professional and public concern with the effect of the total environment in health. *Note* The terms build on the old . . . public health which struggled to tackle health hazards in the physical environment . . . It now includes the socio-economic environment (for example, high unemployment). 'Public health' has sometimes been used to include publicly provided personal health services, such as maternal and child care. The term new public health tends to be restricted to environmental concerns and to exclude personal health services, even preventive ones such as immunization or birth control.

(Draper, 1991)

This recent definition is controversial, both for its breadth and for its exclusion of formal health services. Not all would agree with this version. It also evokes an historical legacy – which is perhaps a matter of more general agreement. It takes as its reference point the nineteenth century history of public health, the 'heroic' or 'golden age' that provides, so it is argued, an earlier example of environmentalism in action. The spur to reform was epidemic disease and especially the impact of cholera outbreaks in 1831–2, 1848 and again in the 1860s. The 'hero' of the period (if we are writing heroic history) was Edwin Chadwick, and his famous *Report on the Sanitary Condition of the Labouring Population* (1842) (Chadwick 1997). Chadwick drew the link between dirt and disease, and its association with overcrowding and poor sanitation. He called for better water supplies, drainage and sewage removal. As a follower of Jeremy Bentham's Utilitarian creed, he saw a strong role for the central state in order to achieve the greatest good for the greatest number, but Chadwick's practical impact was slight. The Public Health Act of 1848 set up a Central Board of Health but legislation was only permissive and not compulsory – and there was strong opposition to dictatorship from the centre. Chadwick was removed from his post in 1854 and the Board was abolished. In other industrializing states, however, such conflicts were avoided simply by rejecting the expansion of the central state (Porter 1994).

In Britain, it was at the local level that most was achieved. Sir John Simon, as Medical Officer to the Privy Council Office, helped to push through Public Health Acts in 1872 and 1875 which forced every local authority to establish a sanitary body as well as to inspect housing and monitor food supplies and 'nuisances'. His resignation in 1876 diminished central influence – but local activity still proceeded apace. The Medical Officer of Health (MoH), compulsory for the first time at the local level under the 1875 Act, could be a crucial engine of change at the local level (Eyler 1997).

Looking at long-term evaluative trends, there are a number of issues to bear in mind about the nineteenth century story. The first of these is the nature of the links between poverty and ill health. Chadwick was Secretary to the Poor Law Commission and his concern for health reform arose out of the concern for pauperism. Ill health caused poverty and therefore a possible reliance on the parish and poor relief. This was the 'human capital' approach to health reform, a response which has often been replicated since. The term 'social capital' in contemporary health promotion recalls this legacy. Public health reform was a surrogate and replacement in the nineteenth century for more general social reform (Hamlin 1998).

The question of how much impact public health interventions really had also arises. This has been a long running debate among historical demographers that has implications for those who plan and run health services in the contemporary world. The 'McKeown thesis' view that formal medical interventions actually achieved little and rising living standards achieved more has been challenged by a view that gives a greater role for formal public health in the nineteenth century (McKeown and Record 1962, Szreter 1988, Lewis 1991).

It is important to remember, too, how the impetus behind public health was informed by fear. Fear was focused on what was seen as the growth of a 'residuum', a race of degenerates, physically stunted and morally inferior. The residuum was seen as an agent of infection – both of healthy bodies and of the body politic. Dirt was considered to be dangerous at the individual, but also at the political level. This larger ideological climate for reform was connected with the late nineteenth century concern about environmental pollution – the fear of contamination crossed boundaries of social and health concern. It is from this period that we derive our images of the fog-shrouded East End of London.

Bacteriology and personal prevention

In the twentieth century, the ideology of public health changed and its focus narrowed. Winslow, an American public health authority, identified three phases in the development of public health: the first, from 1840–1890 was characterized by environmental sanitation; the second, from 1890–1910, by developments in bacteriology, resulting in an emphasis on isolation and disinfection; and the third, beginning around 1910, by an emphasis on education and personal hygiene, referred to as personal prevention. Take bacteriology first. The discoveries of Koch and Pasteur in the late nineteenth century made public health more important as a profession – it was now possible to pinpoint specific causes of disease, and bacteriology soon came to dominate the public health curriculum. But at another level, these developments moved the focus of attention away from the environment and towards the individual patient as the locus of infection. In fact, some historians have argued that these theories gained widespread acceptability quickly at the political level precisely because they provided such a circumscribed notion of appropriate intervention. Others have drawn attention to how the terminology of germs was used and only gave way to bacteria after the 1880s. Public health practice was often ahead of theory, although a linear model of innovation was presented publicly (Worboys 2000). At the same time, governments took up the issue of social/welfare reform through universal education, pensions, health insurance and school meals, so the barriers between health and social reform became higher and more impermeable.

Some historians and sociologists argue that bacteriology had a negligible effect on the implementation of policy. Its importance lay in preparing the way for the rise of what has been called 'surveillance medicine' (Armstrong 1983). The new public health of the early twentieth century was indeed founded on the concept of 'personal prevention'. This was also a marriage between public health and eugenics (Jones 1986). The political imperative for reform was apparent, especially after the Boer War had revealed the shortcomings of British army recruits and heightened eugenic fears of 'national deterioration' and 'racial decline' but the focus was on the individual – and especially the individual mother. The concept of 'maternal efficiency' was prevalent. Lewis has pointed to the tensions implicit in the way the infant mortality rate was conceived of as a problem of maternal ignorance (Lewis 1980). The death rate was highest in poor inner city slums, where insanitary living conditions prevailed. Yet public health doctors and civil servants tended to see maternal and child health as a question of providing health visitors, personal services and health education. Mothers were encouraged to breastfeed and to achieve higher standards of domestic hygiene. The possibility of rising living standards and real wages during the First World War may have had more impact on the infant mortality rate (Dwork 1987), but public health came increasingly to mean the delivery of personal health services.

Running health services in the interwar years

This focus on the personal and the medical ownership of the area meant that what public health doctors did was less distinctive. How did public health doctors differ from general practitioners? The local authority clinic, home of the Medical Officer of Health, seemed to many general practitioners to be offering only what they could also provide through their individual practices. At the same time, when local government took on the administration of Poor Law hospitals after 1929, many public health doctors found themselves running hospitals. The range of services under the public health umbrella in these interwar years was huge – especially in London, where the municipal hospital system was one of the most extensive in the world. Some argued at the time – and historians have underlined this conclusion – that this administrative expansion was achieved only at the expense of the neglect of the 'community watchdog' role of the Medical Officer of Health. (Webster 1982, Lewis 1991). Increasingly, the cutting intellectual edge of public health lay outside the discipline, in particular through the work of academics in social medicine, who remained distinct from public health practitioners.

Post-war failure and realignment

Public health, contrary to the expectations of many in the profession, did not form the basis of a reformed health service post war. Public health doctors lost their hospital role, and faced a decline in clinic work because of the universal access provided to the general practitioner. The local authority role was also under strain with the desire of parts of the public health empire – sanitary inspectors, social workers – to break away. The notion of 'community medicine', of the public health doctor as health strategist, arose at this time. Jerry Morris at the London School of Hygiene and Tropical Medicine first defined the principles of such work as founded in the principles of epidemiology – the community physician would be responsible for 'community diagnosis' and therefore the effective administration of health services. This was the vision put into practice through the policy documents of the late 1960s – the Seebohm Committee and the Todd Commission on Medical Education. Community physicians were to be the linchpin of the NHS, linking all aspects of lay and medical administration (Lewis 1986). They were to be both advisers and managers. In practice, these roles were difficult to juggle. There were tensions between the responsibility to the community outside the hospital and the accountability to the health authority. After health service reorganization in the 1980s community medicine virtually disappeared (Berridge 2001).

This is a British story, and the detail of these developments was not universally replicated in all countries. Dorothy Porter has pointed out, for example, that industrialization was not a necessary prerequisite for central government intervention in health, nor was the centralization model automatically adopted by states. Forms of public health were clearly dependent on the history and cultures of particular countries (Porter 1994). In general however, changes in the ideology of public health have been similar in both Europe and North America. It is worth stopping briefly at this point to recapitulate some of the themes that emerge from this British-focused history and which have relevance to the rise of health promotion in the last quarter of the twentieth century. The public health mandate has narrowed from broad social reform to individual reformation, while the tension between health promotion and preventive activities in the community has often taken second place to a focus on health services and especially their planning and evaluation. Public health personnel/doctors seem to have fallen more readily into the technician-manager rather than the community watchdog role. The relationship with the structures of clinical medicine – as public health has become a medical profession – has been an additional complicating factor.

The 'contemporary history' of health promotion policies

So this leads us naturally into the second level of historical evaluation, the rationale behind the emergence of a new variant of public health called health promotion. Here the post-war shift from infectious to chronic disease as a major cause of ill health and mortality led to an increased emphasis on prevention. Prevention was not an environmental issue, but rather a question of remedying defects in individual lifestyle. The rise of this style of thinking can be traced both internationally and nationally, through for example the 1974 Lalonde report. Many countries followed in publishing similar prevention-oriented documents and there was a rapid growth of interest in preventive medicine and in health promotion. The roots of this reorientation can be traced to the research in the 1940s and 1950s that linked smoking with the rise in lung cancer. These scientific 'discoveries', so historians have argued, represented a fundamental 'paradigm shift' in scientific 'ways of knowing'. For biomedical theories of direct causation they substituted the epidemiological notion of 'relative risk' and statistical correlation (Brandt 1990). Within the discipline of statistics, bio-metrics gave place to public health epidemiology. Epidemiology became the new public health/preventive discipline par excellence, associated with a whole host of health issues, from alcohol and smoking through to diet and heart disease (Blane, Brunner and Wilkinson 1996). This was the epitome of the surveillance society. A public health agenda emerged in the 1960s and 1970s that was based on individual avoidance of risk. It developed a strong economic dimension (the 'human capital' arguments of the nineteenth century revisited), and a focus on education of the individual. Consequently the role of health education assumed new significance alongside the use and development of techniques of mass persuasion in the health area. These also drew on parallel developments in educational practice in particular in relation to developing countries.

Criticism of this approach came from a variety of directions. Some saw the emphasis on individual responsibility for health as a political ploy to divert attention from the real socio-economic causes of disease and the failures of health care systems (Tesh 1981). These condemned the 'victim blaming' and 'sickness as sin' arguments implicit within preventive health. The individual responsibility argument divorced the person from the social environment. This type of argument was demonstrated by the increasing focus in anti-smoking campaigns on the role of women as mothers (a classic historic public health theme) – a naked smoking mother was portrayed in Saatchi and Saatchi advertisements of the 1970s. Mothers were condemned, via epidemiological research, for the low birthweights of their babies, and even for the reduced attainment of their children in later life. There was little sensitivity to the cultural and social realities of life for many women.

Criticism came also from an entirely different direction – from the radical right, which argued that government wished to institute what it called the 'nanny state' where habits which should be left to individual discretion were regulated and controlled unnecessarily (Le Fanu 1994). Proponents of this line of argument often called attention to the fragility of the scientific arguments supporting particular preventive policies. Prevention was crucially about the reduction of statistical risk to the community as a whole, not, as in curative medicine, about delivering benefits to identifiable individuals. In surveys where the public ranked different medical and health interventions, medical technology ranked high while lifestyle efforts received lower levels of public support.

In the post-war years, it was the smoking issue that most clearly epitomized the reorientation of public health towards individual lifestyle. By the 1970s, anti-smoking interests had developed a policy agenda that focused on economic argument (price and tax rises, anti-industry) and on the media (advertising bans, mass media campaigns), sustained through the techniques of epidemiology (Berridge 2003). In the 1980s, the development of AIDS as an issue also epitomized many of those public health concerns. AIDS was a syndrome initially defined solely via epidemiology and through the concept of risk. In the debate on how to respond to the potential epidemic, the old punitive responses of public health to infectious disease – quarantine and notification – were explicitly rejected, often on the advice of historians. AIDS was an epidemiological syndrome par excellence; and it also seemed to exemplify the key tenets of the new public health, stressing individual behaviour modification and individual responsibility rather than any collective reaction (Berridge 1996, Leichter 1991). In the policy responses favoured by western liberal democracies – behaviour modification and health education campaigns – it exemplified the tenets of health promotion.

Recently, new variants of health promotion have emerged. Political change has brought the issue of inequalities back onto the agenda (Berridge and Blume 2003) and other themes are allied to the new environmentalism. Again the precise meaning and content is unclear. The global environment is involved, but also a redefinition and expansion of risk at the level of the individual in society, the concept of the environmental citizen, a rational consumer protecting him or herself from environmental risks (Petersen and Lupton 1996). Health promotion/public health seems to exemplify a new environmental individualism, epitomized by the emergence of the concept of passive smoking, which gave the epidemiological concept of risk an environmental dimension, but one still rooted in the control of individual behaviour and with a strong moral component. Environmentalism at the level of the city or the locality means essentially control of the individual, as for example through the concept of community safety and its elaboration in drug- and alcohol-free spaces. Reforming environmentally damaging social activities is a major thrust of this new health promotion environmentalism.

The history of evaluation

So far we have looked at the meaning of historical analysis in the evaluation of health promotion. But we can also turn the issue on its head and ask – why are we talking about evaluation at all? If we went back say thirty or forty years, not only would we not be talking about health promotion as a concept, we would not be thinking of evaluation as one either. Evaluation is also a historically contingent concept and activity. Why is it now so important? To answer that question would take longer than current space allows – and in fact, no contemporary history of evaluation has been written. A few salient issues can briefly be sketched in. Clearly the rise and reorientation of statistical thinking in the post-war years -through epidemiology and the randomized controlled trial – provided an important mind set for this type of approach. Another strand came via the US 'war on poverty' programmes of the 1960s and, in developing countries, via donor-funded primary health care initiatives. For both, evaluation had political value in demonstrating 'what worked' and in providing the rationale for further funding. In Britain, a key text so far as health services were concerned was Archie Cochrane's 1971 book *Effectiveness and Efficiency*, which presented powerful arguments for the widespread use of the randomized controlled trial in health services (Cochrane 1971) (see Chapter 5). This, he felt, would open up 'a new world of evaluation and control which will, I think, be the key to a rational health service'. Cochrane's specific arguments need to be set in the context of changes in research policy in the 1970s in Britain.

The Rothschild 'customer/contractor' reforms in the funding of research by government departments saw much greater potential government planning of research and control over what researchers did. In the health field, the emergence of the evidence-based medicine movement in the 1980s used primarily statistical and economic techniques (see Chapter 4) to decide if interventions were effective. Such approaches were at the basis of the NHS Research and Development programme launched in the 1980s. Increasingly, these arguments were applied across the health arena to preventive as well as curative interventions. Researchers debated whether prevention was cost-effective, arguing, for example, that stopping smoking could increase costs through greater demands on pensions and welfare benefits by people who lived longer as a result. The methodology of the randomized controlled trial (see Chapter 5), increasingly synonymous with 'evidence' (as if there were no other forms of evidence) in health services, also began to be advocated for health promotion interventions. One reason for this was the close relationship between 'treatment' and preventive interventions. Treatment in many instances was defined as almost synonymous with public health. The technique, originally used in medicine to evaluate the use of new drugs, spread to preventive interventions in areas such as smoking. Many researchers were uneasy about its inexorable rise, citing its origins in the disciplines of the natural and biological sciences and doubting its universal applicability to programmes as opposed to treatments. Underpinning all these developments was the belief, disputed by some, that rationality could indeed be achieved in health policy and in the nature of interventions. Evaluation and evidence-based policy assumed a depoliticized and atomized health arena. It was noticeable that evaluations rarely incorporated the activities of central government (Berridge 2005).

Historical evaluation

Historical evaluation of health promotion, as should be clear from this brief survey, does not set out to give some of the answers traditionally associated with the process of evaluation. It cannot tell us what works best, what is cost-effective, which intervention to put in place, or advise us on the best technique for assessment. Rather this chapter has tried to point out how health promotion is the latest variant of a public health history that traces its origins to the desire of states to deal with issues of social order and control. It has examined, too, how its current ideology has developed out of the changes in public health concepts which have taken place since the nineteenth century, but in particular since 1945. Health promotion should drop its current tendency to focus on and idealize the nineteenth century for its 'lessons'. It should also examine its post-1945 history and why that has emphasized behavioural rather than structural explanations.

Key points

♦ The mandate of public health has redefined itself since the nineteenth century – from environmentalism to personal prevention, to running health services, and on to the focus on individual lifestyle and 'risk'.

♦ Such redefinitions have been inextricably connected with changes in the perceived role of the state and the nature and forms of social order.

♦ The new environmentalism of contemporary health promotion can be seen as a type of environmental individualism, a refocusing of the lifestyle arguments to encompass sites of risk.

♦ The notion of evaluation itself in relation to medicine, health and latterly health promotion is historically contingent. Policy development has rarely been the rational process implied.

♦ Using the nineteenth century as a 'golden age' support mechanism for contemporary policy risks misunderstanding both past and present. Historical analysis can help in assessing current ideologies and policies. To do that, it needs to examine more recent health promotion history.

References

Armstrong, D. (1983) *Political Anatomy of the Body. Medical knowledge in Britain in the twentieth century.* Cambridge University Press, Cambridge.

Berridge, V. (1996) *AIDS in the UK: the making of policy, 1981–1994.* Oxford University Press, Oxford.

Berridge, V. (2001) Jerry Morris. *International Journal of Epidemiology,* **30,** 1141–1145.

Berridge, V. (2003) Post war smoking policy in the UK and the redefinition of public health. *Twentieth Century British History,* **14** (1), 61–82.

Berridge, V. and Blume, S. (eds) (2003) *Poor Health. Social inequality before and after the Black Report.* Frank Cass, London.

Berridge, V. (ed.) (2005) *Making Health Policy; Networks in Research and Policy since 1945.* Rodopi, Amsterdam.

Blane, D. Brunner, E., and Wilkinson, R. (1996) The evolution of public health policy: an anglocentric view of the last fifty years. In D. Blane *et al.* (eds) *Health and Social Organization Towards a health policy for the twenty-first century,* pp. 1–17. Routledge, London.

Brandt, A. (1990) The cigarette, risk and American culture. *Daedalus,* Fall issue, 155–176.

Chadwick, E. (1997) *Report on the sanitary condition of the labouring population of Great Britain 1842 with a new introduction by David Gladstone.* London Routledge/Thoemmes Press.

Cochrane, A. (1971) *Effectiveness and efficiency. Random reflections on health services.* London Nuffield Provincial Hospitals Trust.

Dwork, D. (1987) *War is Good for Babies and Other Young Children. A history of the infant and child welfare movement in England, 1898–1918.* Tavistock, London.

Draper, P. (1991) *Health through Public Policy: the greening of public health.* Greenprint, London.

Eyler, J. (1997) *Sir Arthur Newsholme and State Medicine, 1885–1935.* Cambridge University Press, Cambridge.

Hamlin, C. (1998) *Public Health and Social Justice in the age of Chadwick. Britain, 1800–1854.* Cambridge University Press, Cambridge.

Jones, G. (1986) *Social Hygiene in Britain.* Croom Helm, London.

Le Fanu, J. (1994) *Preventionitis. The exaggerated claims of health promotion.* Social Affairs Unit, London.

Leichter, H. (1991) *Free to be Foolish. Politics and health promotion in the United States and Great Britain.* Princeton University Press, Princeton, NJ.

Lewis, J. (1980) *The Politics of Motherhood. Child and maternal welfare in England, 1900–1939.* Croom Helm, London.

Lewis, J. (1986) *What Price Community Medicine?* Harvester, Brighton.

Lewis, J. (1991) The origins and development of public health in the UK. In W Holland *et al.* (eds) *The Oxford Textbook of Public Health*, 2nd edn, pp. 23–33. Oxford University Press, Oxford.

McKeown, T. and Record, R. G. (1962) Reasons for the decline of mortality in England and Wales during the nineteenth century. *Population Studies*, **xvi**, 94–122.

Petersen, A. and Lupton, D. (1996) *The New Public Health. Health and self in an age of risk.* Sage, London.

Porter, D. (1994) *The History of Public Health and the Modern State.* Rodopi, Amsterdam.

Szreter, S. (1988) The importance of social intervention in Britain's mortality decline, c. 1850–1914: a reinterpretation of the role of public health. *Social History of Medicine*, **1** (1), 1–37.

Tesh, S. (1981) Disease, causality and politics. *Journal of Health Politics, Policy and Law*, **6** (3), 369–390.

Webster, C. (1982) Healthy or hungry thirties? *History Workshop Journal*, **13**, 110–129.

Worboys, M. (2000) *Spreading Germs. Disease theories and medical practice in Britain, 1865–1900.* Cambridge, University Press, Cambridge.

Part II

Methods of evaluation

Chapter 3

Evaluating according to purpose and resources
Strengthening the evidence base incrementally

Yolande Coombes

Evaluation uses a variety of resources including financial, technical, human, time and knowledge (or evidence). All too often the lack of resources leads to a situation whereby evaluation is abandoned because the gold standards of experimental designs cannot be attained, and in the process a lot of useful information which could also contribute to strengthening the evidence base for health promotion is lost or over-looked. Our desire for quick fixes and rapid improvement means that there is tendency to want evaluations that answer definitive questions with certainty. However, it is important to remember that evidence in any field rarely comes from just one source, and often the smallest pieces of evidence incrementally add up to the strongest case. We must be careful that in our search for evidence and the need to evaluate that we do not confuse small-scale or incremental evaluation with poor evaluation.

The need to evaluate

In the introduction to this book we put forward the reasons for the ever-increasing importance placed on evaluation:

- Emphasis on the concepts of efficiency and cost-effectiveness central to development of new initiatives;
- The importance of quality assurance and audit;
- The need for health promotion to engage credibly with the evidence-based medicine movement.

Over the past few years there has been an associated increase in the discussion in the literature about the development of an evidence base for health promotion (Raphael 2000, Davies and MacDonald 1998, Nutbeam 1999) and WHO has endorsed a resolution supporting the 'development of evidence-based health promotion policy and practice within the organization' (WHO 1998). There can be no doubt about the importance of the role of evaluation and its contribution to the creation of a sound evidence base for health promotion.

Strengthening the evidence base for health promotion

The main problem we face in determining the evidence base for health promotion is deciding what counts as evidence. It can be argued that part of the problem that we face in health promotion comes from the difference in how health promotion and health itself are defined and how their impact is measured. Health in the context of health promotion is usually defined in such terms as 'a resource for everyday living' or 'complete mental, physical, spiritual and emotional well-being, not just the absence of disease'; yet evidence is usually taken in the form of a reduction in mortality or morbidity (Raphael 2000). The social, economic and emotional determinants of health are often overlooked in the search for evidence for effectiveness that fit a more biomedical approach to health and health promotion. McQueen (2001) suggests that evidence in health promotion does not really come from health promotion as a discipline itself, but from the effectiveness of a disciplinary subcomponent of the health promotion intervention. This leads to health promotion being reduced to its component parts and rarely being evaluated in a holistic sense – which is how the discipline defines itself.

Yet the holistic nature of health promotion is one of its key strengths. A report produced for the European Commission on the evidence of health promotion effectiveness identified a considerable body of evidence (IUHPE 1999). This report concluded that:

1 Comprehensive approaches using all five Ottawa strategies: public policy; supportive environments; personal skills; community action; and health services are the most effective.

2 Certain settings such as schools, workplaces, cities and local communities offer more practical opportunities for effective health promotion.

3 People – including those most affected by health promotion issues – need to be at the heart of health promotion programmes and the decision-making process to ensure real effectiveness.

4 Real access to information and education in appropriate language and styles is vital.

5 Health promotion is a key investment – an essential element of social and economic development.

In addition Raphael (2000) argues that enough evidence exists to justify health promotion as a discipline that can improve the health of the population and that there is also enough evidence concerning the impact of the determinants of health (biomedical, structural or lifestyle). He therefore argues that what is needed is more accumulated evidence of evaluation of programs and interventions at the local level to see whether they have been effective. Tones (1997) argues that instead of trying to achieve evidence from one source we should follow the format of a judicial review where we can accept evidence even where 100% proof is not available. Combining these two points suggests the need for more evaluations at all levels, focused on particular contexts. There will always be a role for large-scale evaluation studies to prove beyond doubt the efficacy of particular interventions, but evidence takes many forms and the applicability and effectiveness in the local context should not be overshadowed.

McQueen (2001) cites the Centre for Disease Control Guide (2000) in which the definition of the term evidence for health promotion includes:

1 Information that is appropriate for answering questions about an intervention's effectiveness.

2 The applicability of effectiveness data (i.e. the extent to which available effectiveness data is thought to apply to additional populations and settings).

3 The intervention's positive or negative side effects.

4 Economic impact.

5 Barriers to implementation of interventions.

This is not to say that an evaluation must cover all these five points, but that each or all of them contribute to the evidence base. A small-scale evaluation concentrating on the process of implementation and a focus on effectiveness provides a contribution to the evidence base just as a large-scale efficacy trial provides a contribution. The difference is the level of contribution and the focus of the intervention, but ultimately both contribute (see Chapter 5 for a discussion on efficacy versus effectiveness). Just as the level of evidence is important, so too is ensuring that the intervention selected is appropriate for the health problem and, following on from that, that the evaluation method is appropriate for the intervention (Nutbeam 1999). Nutbeam goes on to say (p. 100):

> The most compelling evidence of effectiveness comes from studies that combine different research methodologies – quantitative and qualitative. The use of a diverse range of data and information sources will provide more relevant and sensitive evidence of the effects of multi-dimensional health promotion interventions than a single 'definitive' study.

Nutbeam argues that given the complexity of health promotion interventions and thus their evaluations there can be no 'absolute' form of evidence as is seen in the biomedical sciences and no 'right' method of evaluation. He suggests that evidence for effectiveness is linked to the entry point of the evaluation and the intervention. McQueen (2001) echoes this by saying that as the complexity of an intervention increases we need more complicated methods of assessment, and that answers provided by that assessment may be less clear. He notes that the most rigorous method of assessment, the randomized controlled trial (RCT), is most suited to simple interventions.

However, the move to establishing a sound evidence base for health promotion is associated with an increased focus on outcomes and therefore the need for outcome evaluation. Outcome evaluation needs more resources to get the precision needed for hard or more distal outcomes. The RCT is sometimes put forward as the gold standard for producing reliable evidence. However even the RCT has limitations (see Chapter 5), particularly within health promotion where random allocation of individuals or communities to experimental and control groups is not always possible. Green and Tones (1999 p. 134) note that

> Health promotion is frequently a multifactoral intervention having a range of possible outcomes. Experimental designs that would fully accommodate this intricacy, with the capacity to discriminate between different components of the intervention, would inevitably be highly complex, involve sophisticated analytic techniques, very large samples – and ipso facto, exceed the budgetary constraints of most programmes.

They go on to point out the inadequacy of relying on changes in morbidity and mortality as outcome measures. Their argument is that health promotion interventions should only be developed if they are based on existing evidence that the intervention will have an impact on morbidity or mortality. Morbidity and mortality impact data provide the justification for developing health promotion interventions and not the means of evaluating their effect, particularly at small-scale or local intervention levels.

Evaluating outcome measures over time

It is important to remember that outcome measures change over time. Nutbeam (1998) discusses the concept of outcome hierarchies that emphasize the difference between short-term impact and longer term health outcomes. At one end of the scale immediate measures of effectiveness are characterized by changes in knowledge or skills of individuals, but the scale moves through changes in the determinants of health, health behaviours and socio-economic and environmental conditions to changes in health outcomes in terms of morbidity and mortality at the far end.

Green and Tones (1999) also use this concept of indicators of success along a continuum and point to changes in proximal indicators as being more likely to be due to the impact of the intervention than changes in distal indicators which may take many years to develop. They give the example of 40 years or so for a school-based smoking cessation programme to have an effect on the incidence of lung cancer. They therefore reject epidemiological indicators for evaluating health promotion and instead say the focus of attention should be on the psychosocial

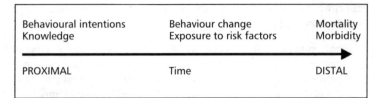

Fig. 3.1 Outcome measures changing over time

and environmental influences on health and health-related decision making. We have an increased theoretical understanding of these influences from a number of explanatory models. They suggest that the use of these models allows the various stages along the continuum from proximal to distal to be defined, and those most proximal to be selected for evaluation (see also Chapter 7). Figure 3.1 outlines how we might examine different outcome measures over time.

The advantage of this continuum perspective is that where links between indicators at different points on the continuum have already been evaluated and established there is no need demonstrate the relationship again, and therefore our evaluation efforts should be concentrated on the relationships between indicators where the evidence is less well established (Green and Tones 1999).

Example

Population Services International are running a campaign across several countries in East and Southern Africa to increase personal risk perception of HIV/AIDS with the aim of increasing safer sex behaviours. This campaign seeks to increase caution and received assurances between partners (such as agreeing on mutual faithfulness or going for Voluntary Counselling and Testing [VCT]) but maintain interpersonal trust whilst reducing sexual trust. We already know that safer sex behaviour is related to a cluster of psychological, social and environmental influences including: beliefs about benefits outweighing barriers; self-efficacy and the ability to negotiate

Example *(Contd.)*

condom use or partner assurances; availability of condoms and personal risk perception. The PSI programme is therefore being evaluated by reporting changes in these indicators in addition to changes in trust, caution and received assurances at the proximal end of the evaluation continuum. Further along the continuum, reported sexual behaviour will be evaluated including reduction in partners, consistent condom use and uptake of VCT. The furthest distal changes in incidence of HIV sero-conversion will not be evaluated as these will be too difficult to attribute to the campaign and will take a long time to measure, they will also be subject to too much background 'noise' from other interventions and campaigns.

Evidence can be built incrementally. Our goal is to reduce the incidence and prevalence of HIV/AIDS and we know this can be done through reducing the number of sexual partners, abstinence, mutual faithfulness and consistent condom use. We already have the evidence on some of the determinants of safer sex behaviour (as outlined above). Therefore to evaluate the intervention we do not need to evaluate distal reductions in morbidity or mortality, or even reductions in incidence or prevalence. The evaluation can be at the proximal end of the continuum by demonstrating changes in personal risk perception (as measured by trust, caution and received assurances) and associated changes in exposure to risk factors and behaviour change.

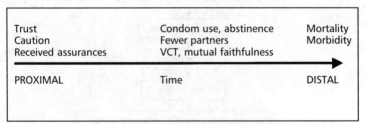

Trust Caution Received assurances	Condom use, abstinence Fewer partners VCT, mutual faithfulness	Mortality Morbidity
PROXIMAL	Time	DISTAL

Fig. 3.2 Outcome measures for the PSI personal risk perception/trusted partner campaign

Each point on the continuum of outcome evaluation needs different indicators of measurement. To decide what these indicators are and what the nature of the evaluation should be we first need to answer the question – Why are we evaluating? Habicht *et al.* (1999) argue that this question is seldom discussed yet is fundamental to choosing an appropriate evaluation design. They suggest that the main objective of any evaluation is to influence decisions, therefore how complex and precise an evaluation is needed is dependent on who the decision-maker is and on what types of decisions will be taken as a consequence of the findings. Both complex and simple evaluations should be equally rigorous in relating the evaluation design to the decisions. These arguments are similar to Andreasen's backwards research process, which was originally developed for market research (see Figure 3.3). The backwards research process is based on the premise that a researcher should first decide what decisions are going to be taken on the basis of the research findings and work backwards from that point to design research (see Chapter 7).

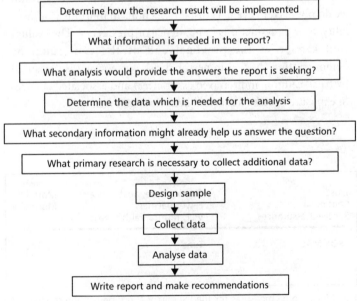

Fig. 3.3 The backwards research process

For the purpose of evaluation Andreasen's (1985) backwards research process can be combined with Habicht *et al.*'s (1999) framework for outcome evaluation. The framework is based on two classification axes. The first axis refers to the indicators in terms of whether they measure the performance of the intervention delivery or its impact on health or behavioural indicators. The second axis refers to the type of inference or attribution that can be made about the intervention and the level at which this should be done. They describe the three levels as adequacy, plausibility or probability.

The adequacy level assesses whether the expected changes occurred. Evaluation at this level is the cheapest and easiest form of evaluation. It does not require the use of control group data as long as results are compared to preset criteria. However if trends in adequacy are to be measured over time then at least two measurements will be required, increasing the complexity of the evaluation. It is not possible to link adequacy measures to intervention outcomes but they can provide reassurance that expected goals are being met. This leads us back to the question of why the evaluation is being carried out. If the decision to be taken on the basis of the evaluation is about whether to continue support for a programme, then adequacy assessment may be all that is needed.

At the level of plausibility assessment the question should be framed in terms of 'Did the intervention seem to have an effect above and beyond other external influences?'. Plausibility assessment is needed where the decision-makers require a greater degree of confidence that observed changes were in fact due to the intervention. Plausibility assessment requires rigorous study designs to control for confounding by external factors that might have influenced changes. Finally at the level of probability assessment, the answer to the question 'Did the intervention have a statistically significant effect?' is being sought. Evaluation at this level needs far more rigorous research design utilizing RCT or longitudinal study designs.

Although Habicht *et al.*'s (1999) framework is useful for determining the level of outcome and impact evaluation, it does not include an analysis of process evaluation (see Chapter 6). Process evaluation is an essential component of any impact or outcome evaluation or can be an evaluation in itself. We might place process evaluation (as an end in itself) as one level lower than adequacy assessment, but also as a component of adequacy, plausibility and probability assessment criteria for our evaluation. A model of the backwards evaluation process would then look like Figure 3.4.

In summary, evaluation in terms of outcomes can take place on a continuum. The evidence we already have on the relationship between different indicators on that continuum determines the level of our outcome evaluation. Second, our level of evaluation should be focused on what decisions will be taken on the basis of the evaluation – this helps us to determine whether adequacy, plausibility or probability evaluation is needed, and thus feeds into the evaluation design. As is noted throughout this book, it is essential to design the evaluation at the outset of the intervention to determine the nature and type of evaluation and the associated resources that will be needed. However, it is possible that following this backwards evaluation process, even at the planning stage, might lead to the conclusion that there are not enough resources to carry out the required level of evaluation. What then? The tendency in this case is sometimes to forego any evaluation, and thus to deny any further contributions to the evidence base.

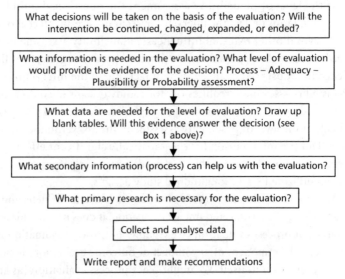

Fig. 3.4 The backwards evaluation process

Evaluation in resource-poor settings

Some would argue that unless an evaluation can be carried out an intervention should not be implemented. However, this contradicts what we have already established – that there is already a strong evidence base in health promotion. Therefore there are many interventions that do not need to be rigorously evaluated by health outcomes. We should be rolling out an intervention once its efficacy and effectiveness have been established. In these situations, evaluation can centre on process and implementation issues and these can be carried out even with minimal resources. If the design and implementation of an intervention are well documented and good cost and activity data are kept, then an intervention can be evaluated in comparison with other interventions, including those that provided the evidence of effectiveness. It all goes back to the question – what decisions will be taken on the basis of the evaluation?

The costs and resources for evaluation can also be minimized by utilizing other routinely collected data or secondary data sources and supplementing this with a process evaluation. Proper documentation of process also allows for the possibility of a retrospective evaluation at a later date.

Conclusion

The evidence base for health promotion is increasing all the time. There is a tendency to try to evaluate outcomes at the highest level in order for them to be considered 'evidence'. However, evidence can also be pieced together incrementally, and there is a significant role for evaluations that are focussed on specific contexts for implementation. Outcome evaluation can occur on a continuum and interventions can focus their evaluation on those outcomes closest to the intervention, especially where there is already evidence for the existence of a relationship between indicators on that continuum. The key question to be asked is how will the evaluation be used – what is its purpose and what decisions will be made? By following a backwards evaluation process we can conserve our resources and aim for an evaluation that will answer the required questions and contribute to the evidence base. Finally, even when resources do not permit outcome evaluation, process evaluation in its simplest forms can help to improve the intervention and can still contribute to the evidence base.

Key points

- Evidence for the effectiveness of health promotion already exists.

- The evidence base can be contributed to from small-scale process evaluations through to randomized controlled trials (RCTs) focused on distal health outcomes.

- Health promotion interventions should be based on existing evidence that the intervention will have an impact on morbidity or mortality as opposed to using morbidity and mortality as a means of evaluating their effect.

- Outcomes occur on a continuum, we can focus an evaluation on proximal indicators where we already have evidence for a relationship between other indicators on the continuum and distal outcomes.

- To design our evaluation we must first ask how the evaluation will be used and work backwards from the answer.

- Even in resource poor settings, small-scale documentation of the process can contribute to the incremental growth of the evidence base.

References

Andreasen, A. R. (1985) Backward market research. *Harvard Business Review*, May/June, 176–182.

Center for Disease Control (2000) Introducing the guide to community preventive services: Methods, first recommendations and expert commentary. *American Journal of Preventive Medicine*, **18** (supplement), 35–43.

Davies, J. and MacDonald, G. (1998) Quality, Evidence and Effectiveness in Health Promotion: Striving for Certainties. Routledge, London.

(IUHPE) International Union for Health Promotion and Education (1999) *The Evidence for Health Promotion Effectiveness: a report for the European Commission by the International Union for Health Promotion and Education.* ECSC–EC–EAEC, Brussels and Luxembourg.

Green, J. and Tones, K. (1999) Towards a secure evidence base for health promotion. *Journal of Public Health Medicine,* **21** (2), 133–139.

Habicht, J. P., Victora, C. G., and Vaughan, J. P. (1999) Evaluation designs for adequacy, plausibility and probability of public health programme performance and impact. *International Journal of Epidemiology,* **28**, 10–18.

McQueen, D. V. (2001) Strengthening the evidence base for health promotion. *Health Promotion International.* **16** (3), 261–268.

Nutbeam, D. (1998) Evaluating health promotion – progress, problems and solutions. *Health Promotion International* **13**, 27–43.

Nutbeam, D. (1999) The challenge to provide evidence in health promotion. *Health Promotion International,* **14** (2), 99–101.

Population Services International. Trusted Partner Campaign funded by AIDSMARK. (personal communication).

Raphael, D. (2000) The question of evidence in health promotion. *Health Promotion International,* **15** (4), 355–367.

Tones, K. (1997) Beyond the randomized controlled trial: a case for a judicial review. *Health Education Research,* **12**, 1–4.

World Health Organization (1998) Resolution of the Executive Board of the WHO on health promotion. *Health Promotion International,* **13**, 266.

Chapter 4

Economic evaluation of health promotion interventions

Warren Stevens

Economic evaluation is often scorned as an attempt by economists to try to put a price on life, but as health professionals or health researchers we cannot afford to underestimate the importance of cost and consequences. We must be alive to the reality that every time we spend a dollar on treating one person we are by definition reducing the resources available to treat another.

In the field of health promotion, in particular, economic evaluation has the potential to be an important political tool. Health promotion and prevention activities are notoriously underfunded due to historical political power in the traditional medical disciplines and because of the societal tendency to overplay the role of treating the sick as compared to preparing the well for future health.

Economic evaluation can show health promotion interventions in their true light, and in a comparable measure of value with treatments. Measures such as cost per life year saved, cost per Quality-Adjusted Life Year (QALY), or Disability Adjusted Life Year (DALY)* averted have become as relevant as the more traditional outcomes of mortality rates and disease burden. All health interventions are an investment in future health and well-being, and economic evaluation

---

* QALY (Quality-Adjusted Life Year) and DALY (Disability Adjusted Life Year) – common composite measures of the health benefit used in economic evaluation, specifically cost-utility analysis.

has the power to show whether and when health promotion can have a better return than simply waiting for the disease to appear before treating it.

This chapter briefly touches on why we should not expect infinite resources at our disposal, and the theory of optimization of benefits within limited resources. It then goes on to look more practically at measuring costs and benefits, dealing with uncertainty around measurement and the effect of this uncertainty on transferring results from one location to another. There is a case study that looks at the introduction of bed nets in the Gambia and then finally some discussion on some of the more common debates in the field.

Theory into practice

All evaluations should consider costs as well as benefits. Welfare economics tells us that when all individuals maximize their health outcomes then society as a whole has maximized its health outcomes. Given a world of finite resources, our aim to maximize health outcomes is only restricted by the resources we have to achieve this goal.

That is, the cheaper and more beneficial each health care intervention is, the more likely it is to move us towards our society's goal of health maximization. To enable us to make these decisions we need to know how much benefit each intervention can give us for our dollar, so that we allocate our resources such that our health benefits are maximized.

Economics looks at how best to allocate scarce, or limited resources to best satisfy often-unlimited demand. All resources are scarce. No matter how much there is of something it will eventually run out. Economists attempt to maximize aggregate benefit from within the restriction of limited resources. The theory of benefit maximization is best described in terms of allocative, or Pareto, efficiency.

Pareto efficiency was named after the economist who first presented this theory, Vilfredo Pareto. He stated that any redistribution of resources would improve efficiency if it made at least one person better off without making anyone else worse off. Society would, therefore, be most efficient where it is impossible to redistribute resources to make someone better off without simultaneously making someone else worse off. There could be a number of different permutations of resource allocation that resulted in Pareto efficiency, but they would all produce the exact same level of aggregate benefit. This is perfectly acceptable in theory but becomes difficult to measure in practice. For example, how is benefit defined? Do some things benefit some people more than others?

The concept is developed further by the 'compensation principle' introduced by Kaldor (1939) and Hicks (1940). It adds the concept of relative or net benefit, making the model more flexible. If a redistribution of resources results in gainers and losers, it is a move towards Pareto efficiency but only if the aggregate benefits of the gainers outweigh the aggregate costs of the losers. In principle the gainers can then compensate the losers while still achieving a net benefit. Kaldor and Hicks proposed that the measurement of benefit should be directly comparable with the costs of redistribution and, as such, benefits should be given a monetary value.

From welfare economics with the goal of optimizing the distribution of scarce resources and the tenants of the theories of allocative efficiency, we reach the theoretical base for the development of economic evaluation of public services. It is not possible to decide the resource allocation of public services by the market due to its market's imperfect nature. The allocation of resources therefore requires direct intervention by government, with the goal of maximizing health benefits within the limitations of the scarce resources available to it.

General concepts

Having decided upon our goal of welfare maximization, through funding directed towards the most cost-effective interventions, we now have to address the more practical issue of how best to achieve this. Cost-effectiveness is a simple concept, measuring the benefits from a chosen intervention against the costs borne by undertaking it. However, this simple concept must take place in a complex world, where there are many contradictory factors that will impact on both the outcomes and costs of an intervention. Often complete measurement of costs and effects is impossible, and what has emerged is a science that measures cost-effectiveness in graduations, based on the degree to which it is practical to measure them.

Cost-effectiveness is often used as a catch-all phrase but is simultaneously one of three (or four) 'types' of economic evaluation, which are all peas from the same pod. At one time or another you will hear of cost–benefit, cost–utility or cost-minimization (sometimes called cost-neutral) analyses, as well as the better-known cost-effectiveness. These terms only really differentiate the basic premise in terms of how they measure outcomes, and to what purpose. Cost–benefit analysis attempts to answer the question of whether an intervention is worth investing in by measuring both costs and benefits in one currency, that of money. It relies on creating or calculating a monetary value of both the health benefits as well as the costs, so that a conclusion can be made based on the simplicity of whether one side is greater than the other. Cost-effectiveness analysis on the other hand steps back from valuing outcomes in monetary terms and instead show results as a ratio of costs and benefits. Benefits are measured in a host of composite or proxy measures, such as life years gained or QALYs.

The roots of the economic evaluation method is cost–benefit analysis (CBA), the aim of which is to measure the effect of changes in resource allocation in terms of the net benefit to society. Difficulties arise in the development of methods to measure 'benefit'. However, a version of cost-effectiveness analysis (CEA), known as cost–utility analysis (CUA) attempts to overcome this problem by using a common measure of outcome, so the relative cost-effectiveness of all interventions can be compared. In CUA the benefits are expressed in terms of QALYs, DALYs or the more recent Healthy Year Equivalents (HYEs). These CUA methods can then be used to compare interventions with different outcomes.

Although CBA is the original method of economic appraisal, decision-makers now prefer CEA because it does not require the translation of health consequences into monetary units (i.e. quantifying the value of human life). However, there have been signs recently of a re-emergence of CBA (Diener *et al.* 1998), with the introduction of a number of new methods that have made the valuation of health consequences less problematic. CUA continues to be the fastest growing of the types of economic evaluation, although there is an ongoing debate about the use and calculation of the generic measure of benefit, be it QALYs, DALYs or HYEs.

The application of these methods is under continuous review, with no consensus of opinion (Drummond *et al.* 1993). The choice of method is not straightforward. Options may be limited due to the type and quality of the information available, as well as possible restraints on time and resources. The goal must be to maximize what can be achieved and to choose the method most appropriate to the data.

A key issue that must be considered before embarking on an economic evaluation of any kind is the economic viability of economic analysis, i.e. whether it is worthwhile spending resources on the evaluation. The quality or the availability of information for economic analysis may be so poor that it is not efficient to conduct an economic evaluation because the results will be unreliable. Ideally economic evaluation, with its associated costs, should only be undertaken if the benefits of improving efficiency in the use of health care resources outweigh the costs of the evaluation.

Measuring costs and effectiveness

As discussed in the previous section, our different versions of economic evaluation differ, in the most part, in terms of their methods for measuring and aggregating their measurement of outcomes or benefits. The tools and methods used to measures costs across these different methods are, in the main, universal. Nevertheless, nothing is an academic discipline without debate, and measuring true economic cost is no exception. The three major areas of debate in cost measurement are:

1 The perspective from which our measure of cost originates;

2 Intertemporal differences in real cost, or 'discounting'; and

3 International differences in purchasing power, or shadow-pricing.

There are two broad areas of perspective, which are known as the 'provider' and 'society'. The provider perspective is a supply side measure and is used where the results of the evaluation are destined for a specific customer, usually the organization that will need to free up current resources to fund the new intervention. Its objectives are to understand what costs it will have to bear, what potential savings it could make as a result of the intervention, and what improvements in overall health benefit the population it serves will gain.

Alternatively a study measured from a societal perspective must go outside the impact of the immediate provider and attempt to capture all relevant costs that are borne by providers, potential beneficiaries, their families and other coexisting providers, and aggregate all relevant costs and benefits that may accrue across society as a whole – these are often termed indirect costs. It is this method that sticks most closely to the ethos of welfare economics, because to assess the true benefit to society all such benefits and costs should be included. Inevitably, as we move closer to theoretical perfection we are hit harder by the limitations of practicality.

The theoretical basis of discounting, or time preference, relates to the fact that costs and benefits have a higher value now than in the future, and as such future costs and benefits must be discounted against those in the present. This should make intuitive sense as the opportunity to take any benefit now would be preferred to receiving that benefit some time in the future, and similarly any costs would be favoured if they were borne in years to come rather than in the present.

There is much debate in the literature on the necessity and exact value that should be used to discount both costs and benefits (Gravelle and Smith 2001), and where and when they should be used (Walker and Kumaranayake 2002). This is an important area in health promotion because time is such an important component of the value of the ratio components of cost and effectiveness. Whereas costs are mostly incurred in the present, most benefits will be accrued some time in the future. If the discount rate is too high, or too low, this will have a significant effect on the perceived value of the intervention.

Finally we have the issue of differences in international purchasing power – shadow pricing – in different countries. Shadow pricing is the use of world market or border prices of goods or services used as inputs into the intervention, rather than local prices that may be artificially low or high. The reason for this is partly for translation across borders (this will be discussed later), more importantly it is based on the principle of opportunity cost, which is the key principle that defines all costs in economic theory.

For example, if a particular good required for an intervention were locally priced much lower than the world market price, a better use of that resource would be to export it onto the world market and gain additional resources to produce more. So instead of handing out 10 locally made bed nets that cost $1 each, if the world market price is $5, exporting the 10 bed nets would provide resources for 50 bed nets. In reality perfectly competitive markets tend to prevent these situations from occurring, but the prevalence of tariffs and subsidies across borders mean that these shadow prices often occur, and to use local prices would be to under- or overestimate true costs drastically. A good review of the issues and methods can be seen in Dinwiddy and Teal (1996).

Dealing with uncertainty and the transferability of results

If there has been one area in which health economics has made considerable progress over the last 10 years it is dealing with uncertainty. Economics has been accused of lacking scientific rigour in the past. This is most obviously due to the fact that you cannot control perfectly one aspect of human or societal behaviour in order to measure another. Nevertheless, the joining of economics with health has forced economics to give greater consideration to keeping up with the medical statisticians and epidemiologists in showing the robustness of the results of economic evaluations.

Initially cost-effectiveness was measured deterministically, meaning that just one total cost was measured and was then divided by the best estimate of the outcome of interest. As such the robustness of measures of cost-effectiveness were rightly questioned. However, over the last 10 to 15 years, stochastic measures of calculating costs have developed, where multiple estimates of costs are generated relating to specific cases in the same way that estimates of efficacy and effectiveness are drawn. This has led to the development of cost-efficacy spheres, ellipses or ovals, where the area inside the sphere is the equivalent of the confidence interval surrounding the effect size in statistics. More recently these advances have been combined with methods to incorporate the goals of the decision-maker. To achieve this, instead of limiting the analysis of the result to a series of ratios the availability of resources, the cost-effectiveness of alternative interventions and the priorities of the decision-maker are incorporated into the analysis and the results emerge as cost-effectiveness curves (O'Brien and Briggs 2002).

Economics is about optimization, whereas the measurement of health interventions has traditionally been about certainty. The primary goal of the evaluation of health-directed interventions is to ensure that nineteen times out of twenty they work to the benefit of the individual receiving the intervention, whereas economics is more geared towards optimization – as long as more people are made better off than those who are made worse off, a societal gain, or an improvement in welfare, has said to have been achieved. For more on this issue see Stevens and Normand (2004).

In the previous section we touched on shadow pricing and the need to make evaluations a useful source of information outside the limited sphere of the intervention under study. Here we come across the issue of internal versus external validity (see also Chapter 5). As important as it is to get the true costs that relate to the effectiveness of an intervention in any given context it is equally important to understand the efficacy: for example, if we wish to gain more knowledge of the true *effectiveness* of a condom campaign in the Peruvian city of Juliaca, we need to understand more than just the *effectiveness* of a condom campaign in Juliaca. Ideally we would like this study to have given at least insight, but possibly also data, that will lead us to a strong belief about the likely efficacy of such an intervention in other Peruvian cities, the whole of Peru, most South American countries and possibly across the world. There will always be limitations to the value of a study shown to be effective in one location and its relevance to others, but the important thing is to capture and differentiate those things that have this potential. The key word here is transparency: when measuring resources it is important to list resources, local prices and world prices. It is also important to use sensitivity analysis, not just where variables are uncertain but where they are likely to vary across the world.

Example: cost-effectiveness of Insecticide-treated Nets (ITNs) in the Gambia

In 1992 the WHO and the Gambian Government initiated the National Impregnated Bednet Programme (NIBP) as an attempt to reduce the effect of malaria on the population. Local primary health care (PHC) centres across the country were given an insecticide (permethrin) with which people could dip their nets, given free of charge to anyone who turned up at the PHC with a bed net. This was a perfect opportunity to measure the cost-effectiveness of treating bed nets with insecticide.

Methods

As this was a question that both the government of the Gambia and the world at large wanted answered a societal perspective was chosen. The method of choice was a cost-effectiveness study with measures including cost per malaria case avoided and cost per life saved, to make it comparable both with other malaria interventions and with other health interventions on a wider scale.

Costs associated with the evaluation itself were excluded, and the main recurrent costs borne by providers were insecticide, personnel, administration and transport. Capital or set-up costs included

Example: cost-effectiveness of Insecticide-treated Nets (ITNs) in the Gambia (Contd.)

vehicles, buildings for storage, equipment for impregnation, and the sensitization and awareness campaign. The sensitization campaign was treated as a capital cost as its effect lasts for more than one cycle of the intervention.

The consequences of the intervention were measured in both process and health outcomes, such as reductions in morbidity and mortality, effect on school attendance and resource savings both in the health sector and in households themselves. Health sector savings were limited to hospital health centre savings due to reduced incidence of disease, whereas at the household level there were saved treatment costs and indirect savings resulting from less time spent caring for sick children and funerals.

Most of these component parts of the intervention, in particular the nets and insecticide themselves, were not produced domestically, so they were bought and costed at world market prices. Government staff carried out the distribution so salaries were costed as local. Capital costs were discounted at 6% reflecting the prevailing Treasury bill rate minus inflation, which is often assumed to be the cost of investment. When assessing wider societal costs or indirect costs, time lost or saved was measured as an appropriate proportion of gross salaries prevailing in the community at the time of dipping. The time is often important – the ideal time to treat nets is often the time farmers are highly active preparing for the rains.

Results

Results were shown in a series of cost-effectiveness ratios including cost per life year gained, cost per child-year protected and cost per impregnated mosquito net. Multi-way sensitivity analysis was undertaken to test the uncertainties in the study. Costs were deterministic in that the intervention was costed as

Example: cost-effectiveness of Insecticide-treated Nets (ITNs) in the Gambia (Contd.)

a whole, and measured against a series of stochastically estimated outcomes.

The total cost was $91,864, with insecticide the biggest component making up 70% of total recurrent costs, therefore cost of insecticide would be a key component of sensitivity analysis. The estimated number of deaths averted was 41, although there was some geographical variation. Estimated life years gained was 1643 (discounted at 6%, this was 605, at 3% 935), and the number of child years of protection was 19,912. This gives us a cost per death averted of $471; a cost per LYG of $27, and a cost per child year protected was just under $1.

Sensitivity analysis showed that the key component parts of the cost-effectiveness ratios were insecticide costs; discount rates used on health benefits, and treatment rates and costs. Using a cheaper insecticide may reduce programme costs by up to 30%, and have a knock-on effect on cost-effectiveness. Lower treatment cost is also likely to have a significant effect on likely savings, while reducing the discount rate on health outcomes from 6% to 3% would reduce the cost per LYG from $27 down to $16.

Discussion

The key to the potential value of this study is the extent to which it can show the potential of the intervention elsewhere; the issue of transferability of results and external validity. The study uses multiple outcomes and sensitivity analysis and, importantly, points out the likely differences between the setting (the Gambia) and other places where the interventions might be used, and the methods (deterministic) employed. Gambia had a high level of bed net usage, and so reproducing this intervention elsewhere would involve a greater investment in distribution, or in creating greater bed net usage across the population. It also highlights the

> **Example: cost-effectiveness of Insecticide-treated Nets (ITNs) in the Gambia** (Contd.)
>
> difficulties inherent in using the study as a sole source of comparison with other health interventions as the methodologies used differ. Nevertheless it is an informative study and a valuable piece of research (Aikins *et al.* 1998).

Efficiency versus equality: a trade-off?

There is often thought to be a trade-off between maximizing aggregate benefits and attaining an equitable distribution of these benefits across the population as a whole. Efficiency considerations are those relating to allocation of resources; marginal costs and benefits to society as a whole are evaluated in terms of the alternative uses of the resources employed, with no attempt to identify the individuals or households which gain or lose. If overall the benefits exceed the costs there is an efficiency gain to be made by implementing the policy.

This is probably an oversimplification of the issue; nevertheless it is something that should be continually addressed when assessing the relative 'efficiency' of different interventions aimed at the same goal – that of maximizing health outcomes. For example, it is often argued that rather than incorporate more new vaccines into the Extended Programme of Immunization (EPI), supported by WHO and UNICEF, countries should be trying to increase their coverage of existing EPI. Total coverage rates for developing countries mostly fall in the range 50–80%, which leaves a large proportion of the population not benefiting from this disease prevention strategy, so spending scarce resources on new vaccines will simply increase inequality. This argument is compounded by the valid assumption that those who are not reached are often those most likely to benefit from these interventions, such as the poor, the uneducated and those living in the most desolate areas of these countries.

One suggested answer to this quandary has been the use of distribution weights to bias policies and projects towards poorer or more disadvantaged members of society. This method has no lack of detractors with Harberger (1978), using the example of moving ice-cream between desert oases; if the poorer beneficiaries in the receiving oasis have a social weight of four, up to three-quarters of the ice-cream could melt on the way to the second oasis without the project being socially unacceptable. Equality issues are probably better dealt with in resource allocation policy rather than by individual interventions, as this can lead to poor direction of specific interventions and overall welfare loss through potential allocation failures such as double counting. For example, if inequality weighting created an allocation of more resources being directed towards specific geographical areas that suffer greater overall disease or ill-health, and then these areas themselves direct a greater than equitable share of resources to diseases which are believed to be underserved, there is a real chance that relative overfunding could occur within this specific area and other potential areas of need could inadvertently suffer as a result. With the marginal benefits from interventions overfunded dropping rapidly and the marginal benefits of underfunded interventions rising, this can lead to the creation of an growing aggregate welfare loss and a reality of wasted resources.

More theoretical discussions on the trade-off of efficiency and equality often centre on the question, 'Is the problem not one of economics but of the practicalities of measuring true benefits?' In reality those in greatest need are likely to have much higher marginal benefits from any specific intervention related to their need. It therefore becomes much more efficient to direct resources to this population as, if there are greater marginal gains per person, then there are greater aggregate gains to society as a whole. The difficulty with this argument lies in measuring in detail the marginal benefits associated with subgroups. The intent to achieve both efficiency and equality is restricted by the tools available.

In summary, economic evaluation is an invaluable tool in health policy and decision-making around resource allocation priorities. Like all other aspects of evaluation, care must be taken to ensure that methods and the quality of outcome measurement are optimized. When done correctly, economic evaluation alone can show and compare the true value of investment into alternative health promotion and health care interventions.

Key points

♦ Resources are not infinite so decisions must be made as to where resources must be allocated to maximize health benefits.

♦ Economic evaluation can be a powerful tool in distinguishing and proving the true value of health promotion interventions compared to disease treatment.

♦ The method of choice for economic evaluation relies on the question to be answered, the comparison to be made and the data available.

♦ The key to transferability of results is transparency of both methods and results and generous use of sensitivity analysis.

♦ Efficiency and equity are two equally admirable goals, but they can be sought and achieved without compromise to each other.

References

Aikins, M. A., Fox-Rushby, J., D'Allessandro, U., Langercock, P., Cham, K., New, L., Bennett, S., Greenwood, B., and Mills, A. (1998) The Gambina National Impregnated Bednet Programme: Costs, consequences and net cost-effectiveness. *Social Science and Medicine* **46**, 181–191.

Diener, A., O'Brien, B., and Gafni, A. (1998) Health care contingent valuation studies; a review and classification of the literature. *Health Economics*, 7, 313–326.

Dinwiddy, C. and Teal, F. (1996) *Principles of Cost-Benefit Analysis in Developing Countries*. Cambridge: Cambridge University Press.

Drummond, M. F. *et al.* (1993) Standardizing economic evaluation methodologies in health care: practice problems and potential. *International Journal of Technology Assessment in Health Care*, **9**, 26–36.

Gravelle, H. and Smith, D. (2001) Discounting for health effects in cost-benefit and cost-effectiveness analysis. *Health Economist*, **10**, 587–599.

Harberger, AC. (1978) On the use of distributional weights in social cost-benefit analysis. *Journal of Political Economy*, **86**, S87–120.

Hicks, J. (1940) The valuation of the social income. *Economica*, 7, 105–124.

Kaldor, N. (1939) Welfare propositions of economics and interpersonal comparisons of utility. *Economic Journal*, **49**, 549–551.

O'Brien, B. J. and Briggs, A. H. (2002) Analysis of uncertainty in health care cost-effectiveness studies: an introduction to statistical issues and methods. *Stat Methods Med Res*, 11, 455–468.

Stevens, W. and Normand, C. E. (2004) Developing the use of economic evaluation for decision making through recognizing the importance of heterogeneity. *Social Science and Medicine*, 85, 315–320.

Walker, D. and Kumaranayake, L. (2002) Allowing for differential timing in cost analyses: discounting and annualization. *Health Policy Plan*, 17, 112–118.

Chapter 5

Evaluating interventions
Experimental study designs in health promotion

Annie Britton and
Margaret Thorogood

An experimental study is the standard method for evaluating clinical effectiveness. In such a study, a group of people exposed to an intervention is compared with another group who have not been exposed. There are situations in which an experimental approach may not be feasible or appropriate. However, when possible, well designed, controlled experiments provide reliable evidence on the effectiveness of interventions. There are a range of experimental study designs with different advantages and disadvantages; in this chapter we discuss these different designs and how the most appropriate design might be chosen.

The findings of randomized controlled trials (RCTs) are perceived as reliable and valid evidence, and are highly valued in clinical research, but their use in health promotion has been criticized (Speller 1997). There is suspicion about the perceived dominance of a biomedical system of thought which imposes inappropriate rules, addresses inappropriate questions, and fails to take account of the long duration and complex nature of most health promotion interventions. A lack of RCT evidence should not be interpreted as a weakness. Well-conducted non-randomized studies, corroborated by other qualitative evidence, can provide a sound evidence base for health promotion interventions.

In this chapter we discuss some of the strengths and weaknesses of randomized controlled trials and go on to describe some other forms of experimental design that are used in health promotion.

Experimental research

The idea of testing the effectiveness of a treatment by experimentation on humans has been around for a long time. One elegant experiment was carried out as early as 1747 by a ship's surgeon who was looking for a cure for the scurvy which was then a major manpower problem for the Navy – causing more deaths than 'the united efforts of the French and Spanish arms' (Buck *et al.* 1988). James Lind describes how he took twelve sailors with scurvy whose cases were 'as similar as I could get them'. The sailors 'lay together in one place' and had 'one diet common to all'. They were assigned, in pairs, six different medications, including vinegar, cider, sea water, 'elixir vitriol', a mixture including garlic and mustard seed amongst other things, and 'each two oranges and one lemon every day'. The results were dramatic: 'the most sudden and good effects were perceived from the use of the oranges and lemon; one of those who had taken them being at the end of six days fit for duty'. This early example of a clinical trial contained many of the aspects that are still important in the design of health care trials:

- The question to be addressed had *important public health implications.* It is not ethical to carry out research on humans to answer trivial or irrelevant questions.

- More than one treatment was used and the effects were compared. That is, there was a *control group.*

- Lind attempted to choose patients who were similar and to treat them similarly in all other ways except for the treatment being compared in order to eliminate the effect of other factors, such as severity of disease, that might otherwise have affected the result. That is, he tried to match the groups for *confounding factors.*

- The choice of oranges and lemons as a potential cure to be tested was not haphazard, but was based on the observation of non-experimental accounts of scurvy being cured or prevented when citrus fruit was available. That is, the trial was part of a greater body of work, and he had started by carrying out a *review of the already available evidence.*

We do not know if Lind allocated the treatments randomly, but apart from that, this scientific experiment had many features required in a clinical trial today.

Randomized controlled trials

The two essential features of a randomized controlled trial are that at least two interventions are compared, and that people are allocated at random to the different intervention groups.

Example

Researchers in California wanted to find the best way to encourage increased physical activity amongst sedentary people in late middle age. They sought volunteers for the trial in the local community and then randomized the subjects to one of four groups: one was a control group who were simply assessed for fitness, while the other three were given varying advice on taking exercise. Two groups were recommended to undertake home-based exercise, one of high intensity and one of low intensity, while the third group was recommended to join a high intensity group-based exercise plan. At the end of the trial, the researchers concluded that home-based exercise was as effective as group exercise, and that low intensity exercise (such as brisk walking) was as effective as high intensity exercise. The results of trials such as this are important in the development of new strategies to increase activity and improve fitness (King *et al.* 1991).

Randomization is important because it means that any confounding factors, whether or not they had been previously identified, are likely to be equally distributed between the groups. Hence any difference in outcome that is observed can be attributed with more certainty to the difference in the interventions, rather than the effect of confounding. Confounding factors are factors that are linked to both the intervention and outcome and can therefore distort the estimated effect. For example, a common confounding factor is age, which may affect the way someone reacts to an intervention and is also an important risk factor for almost all health outcomes.

The unit of randomization can either be an individual, so each person is randomized, or in can be a group, so that a whole group of people are randomized together, for example patients seen by a particular doctor, residents of a small town. This kind of community randomization is particularly useful when a community-based intervention, for example, a campaign to increase uptake of childhood vaccination, is being tested. Note that community randomization usually increases the sample size required.

It is important that neither the researcher who is allocating the treatment group, nor the person who is being allocated, can predict the allocation. This is called *concealed allocation*, and is done to prevent any possibility of bias arising from either the participant or the researcher preferring one intervention to another.

It is also preferable that both the participants and the researcher(s) are unaware who is receiving which intervention during the trial, so that measuring the outcome cannot be affected. This is called a *double-blind trial*. Such trials are relatively easy to conduct when the treatment is a pill for which an inactive but otherwise identical placebo can be prepared. It is much less easy, and usually impossible, in trials of health promotion interventions. It is more often possible to carry out a *single-blind trial*, where the person measuring the outcome (for example a nurse measuring blood pressure) does not know the allocation.

In evidence-based medicine, there is a hierarchy of reliable evidence, with the results of RCTs or meta-analyses of those trials at the top (see Box 1). This hierarchy is based on an assessment of how much the different study designs may be affected by bias, and therefore on how certain we can be that the observed effects are attributable to the intervention. However, the value of the evidence also depends on how well the study was designed, conducted, analysed and reported. Poor quality RCTs are less useful than well-designed non-randomized studies.

Box 1 Hierarchy of experimental research evidence

Level Source of evidence

I   Systematic reviews and meta-analyses

II Well-designed randomized controlled trials

III Well-designed controlled studies with quasi-randomization

IV Well-designed controlled studies with no randomization

V   Before and after studies

VI Small case reports or studies with no control group

Systematic reviews and meta-analyses

Systematic reviews and meta-analyses are ways of combining the evidence from a lot of different studies. Sometimes individual studies are too small (underpowered) to answer important research questions, and sometimes a collection of different studies draw different conclusions. Systematic reviews put together all the available evidence, having first systematically (without bias) selected the papers that will be included. The aim is to identify the most reliable evidence. In a meta-analysis this is taken a stage further, in that statistical methods are used to combine the results of different studies and give one or more summary statistics.

Example

The Cochrane Tobacco group has provided a meta-analysis of RCTs that looked at the effectiveness of nurses giving advice to people to stop smoking. After systematic searching and applying uniform inclusion criteria, the authors found 22 relevant trials. They carried

Example *(Contd.)*

out a meta-analysis, which included data from over 9,000 study participants, and concluded that advice from a nurse increased the chances of a smoker quitting, with an odds ratio of quitting of 1.50 (95% confidence interval 1.29 to 1.73) (Rice and Stead 2003).

The Cochrane Collaboration is a worldwide network of academics. They prepare, and regularly update, systematic reviews assessing interventions for prevention, treatment and rehabilitation of health problems. The systematic reviews produced by the Collaboration rely predominantly on evidence from randomized controlled trials and there are now well-documented guidelines for those wishing to prepare such reviews (Chalmers and Altman 1995). Reviews from the Cochrane Library are freely available to anyone in the United Kingdom through the National Electronic Library for Health (http://www.nelh.nhs.uk/).

Unique features of health promotion

Rigorous evaluation is important, but that does not mean that a randomized controlled trial is the best method in every circumstance. The aims of health promotion differ in important ways from those of the curative interventions. There are two dimensions of health promotion that should be considered in planning or reviewing experimental studies that evaluate health promotion interventions.

Nature of the intervention

The intervention being tested in a clinical trial usually has a biological basis (for example, drugs, surgery, or physiotherapy). In health promotion, interventions rarely involve direct manipulation of the biological environment. Health promotion interventions are aimed at achieving behavioural change at either an individual or a societal level. This has repercussions for the design of trials, both in terms of the unit that receives the intervention, which could be an individual, a small community, or a whole nation, and in terms of the concepts of placebo comparisons and blinded participants. It is difficult to devise a placebo comparison intervention for a community development intervention, and almost always impossible to blind people to the fact that they have received counselling or some other form of intervention aimed at helping them to change their behaviour.

Health promotion interventions are usually intended to prevent ill health or unhappiness a long way into the future. For example, a community development project which was concerned with improving access to fresh fruit and vegetables, would only be expected to impact on the health of the population over a period of many years, as children grew up, and middle-aged people became elderly, with a more adequate intake of antioxidants. The focus of health promotion on outcomes in the distant future makes evaluation by RCTs difficult. An RCT lasting ten years or more is difficult and expensive to conduct.

When a community level intervention is being evaluated, there is a risk that neighbouring communities that are acting as control groups will adopt the practices of the intervention community. After all, health promotion interventions address important health problems and it is likely that many communities are looking for solutions to the same problems. This *contamination* is hard to prevent or control.

Moreover, a community body, such as a local authority or a health promotion unit, is responsible for implementing many community interventions. It is easy to design a trial that randomizes communities to different intervention groups, but much less easy to gain the agreement of the implementing organization to the concept of randomization, especially if the members of the organization are elected by the communities that they serve.

Nature of the participants

In a health promotion trial, the participants are unlikely to be seeking a solution for their health problem; in fact, it is probable that the subjects do not perceive that they have a health problem. Clinical trials aim to find a way to cure or ameliorate a condition, and in such trials the participants enter the trial with a health problem, from which they hope to find relief. Often, people will describe their motivation for entering such a trial as 'to help find a cure'. This will not be the case in a health promotion RCT, and this will affect recruitment to a trial. The problem of biased recruitment is discussed in the next section.

Validity of trials

Internal and external validity are both important when evaluating the importance of trial findings. The internal validity is a measure of the extent to which the findings are real and not the result of bias. The groups that are compared should be as alike as possible, except for the intervention or treatment under investigation. In well conducted, blinded, randomized controlled trials internal validity is not usually a problem.

When a trial is not blinded, or only single blinded (i.e. participants are aware of their allocation) results could be biased by the effects of participant preferences. Participants often have strong preferences or beliefs about the effectiveness of interventions and this may enhance or reduce their response (possibly through compliance or via a psychological pathways). For example, in a trial of smoking cessation interventions, participants received either counselling for smoking cessation or hypnosis therapy. If an individual has a strong belief in the effectiveness of hypnosis, they may experience an enhanced response if randomized to hypnosis, and a more negative effect if randomized to counselling. It is very difficult to measure the consequences of preference effects (McPherson et al. 1997), but researchers need to be aware of them when planning trials.

External validity is a measure of how generalizable the findings are to a wider population. Individuals who participate in research trials are different to the rest of the population, and this is even more true of health promotion trials. A review of health promotion studies which reported entry characteristics of both participants and non-participants (Britton et al. 1998) found that trial participants were more likely to be younger; to be of higher social status (in terms of income, housing, education and car ownership); and to believe in and adopt a healthier lifestyle in comparison to non-participants. Non-participants included those not invited to participate (for example, people who failed to meet the eligibility criteria) and those who refused. Where participants are found to differ from the rest of the population, the external validity of the study is weakened.

The external validity can also be compromised by the conditions in which a trial is conducted, which are sometimes far removed from real life practice. For example the eligibility criteria may be very strict and 100% compliance may be achieved (Britton *et al.* 1999). Such trials are called *efficacy* trials because they measure the extent to which a specific intervention, procedure or service produces a beneficial result under ideal conditions. Such findings may not be generalizable or repeatable in normal practice. An *effectiveness* or pragmatic trial is one which takes place in a normal practice setting and is therefore subject to the hazards of non-compliance and loss to follow up. The participants may be very heterogeneous and have co-morbidities, but therefore such trials have higher external validity.

Implications for evaluation

Randomized controlled trials clearly have their place in the evaluation of health promotion (Stephenson and Imrie 1998), but may sometimes prove impossible. When this is the case, other forms of experimental evaluation should be considered. These will lose something in internal validity but may gain in external validity. They can be considered in two categories: those where comparison groups can be identified but randomization is not possible; and those where no comparison group can be identified. In either case, developing a good quality research protocol requires careful thought, and, often, some ingenuity.

Whatever the study design used, the understanding and interpretation of the findings will be enriched by using qualitative methods alongside traditional quantitative methods. As is shown elsewhere in this book, qualitative methods have a crucial role to play at the formative stage of an intervention, and can provide important process data. However, such methods are also valuable in interpreting outcome data.

Example

In a recent trial of an intervention to increase fruit and vegetable consumption, qualitative research was carried out before and after participation in the trial to identify barriers to changing diet that were anticipated, and also those that were encountered, and strategies adopted to overcome them. The quantitative analysis showed that plasma antioxidant levels and reported fruit and vegetable intake increased significantly more in the intervention group, but the policy relevance and value of that observation was enriched by the findings of the qualitative work that the increased cost of a change in diet was a relatively intractable barrier, and that other problems such as getting fruit or vegetables when travelling had not been anticipated but were encountered during the trial (John and Ziebland 2004).

There is useful guidance on randomized controlled trials of complex interventions (Medical Research Council 2000), but that only addresses one small part of evaluating such interventions. Many complex health promotion interventions, involve, for example, community mobilization, mass media campaigns and small group interventions and require a wide range of evaluation techniques, which may include one or more trials, but will also include other techniques discussed in this book. Combining the results of all these various evaluations and reaching agreed conclusions requires careful, mutually respectful, multidisciplinary discussions.

Alternative forms of experimental evaluation

Studies with a current comparison group but without randomization

The three most important considerations in such studies are that the study involves enough people or communities to detect the difference that one is expecting to see, that comparison groups are as similar as possible to the intervention group, both with respect to the prevalence of potential confounding factors and with respect to likely external influences on the outcomes, and that the important characteristics of the two groups are measured before the trial starts.

Example

A study was carried out to test the effect of adding fluoride to drinking water. A community in Cheshire, England, made the decision to add fluoride to the water supply, while there were no such plans in the very similar, neighbouring community with low levels of fluoride in the water. A group of dental researchers saw this opportunity to evaluate the effect of fluoride in the water on post-eruptive teeth. A sample of twelve year old children from each of the two areas were examined by a dentist in the year before fluoridation started, and for the following four years. The results showed that the students drinking the fluoridated water had 25% fewer caries at the end of the four years (Hardwick *et al.* 1982).

These studies are not ideal, and should only be considered where randomized controlled trials are not possible. Many such studies have involved only a small number of communities and have provided inconclusive results. Many of the differences in comparison groups may be unknown or not measurable and so risk-adjustment techniques will not be sensitive enough.

Studies with no current comparison group

Sometimes it is not possible to find an appropriate comparison group. This is usually because the intervention being evaluated has extended over a whole population. In this case the best alternative may be for the intervention group to act as their own controls, so that the effect of the intervention is estimated from the observed change over the period of the intervention. This is sometimes described as a *before-and-after study*.

Example

In Thailand, between 1989 and 1991 a rapid increase in the prevalence of infection in female sex workers was noted, from 3.5% prevalence to 15% prevalence. In response, the Ministry of Public Health set up the '100% Condom Campaign' to control the spread of infection. This was a national campaign, so no current control group was available. The initiative was evaluated by a study of a series of five cohorts of army recruits between 1991 and 1995. Between 1991 and 1993 the prevalence of HIV in army recruits ranged between 10% and 13%. By 1995, it had fallen to 7% (Nelson *et al.* 1996).

Before and after studies have many weaknesses, most particularly that they cannot eliminate the effects of any other changes that are occurring over time, and should only be considered when other types of trial are not possible. However, they can sometimes provide the only available evidence of whether or not an intervention was effective.

Randomized controlled trials versus other quantitative evaluations

Box 1 shows a hierarchy of experimental research evidence, with randomized controlled trials near the top. However, health promotion interventions differ from curative interventions and RCTs may not always be the most appropriate study design. It is often stated that non-randomized studies report larger estimates of intervention effects than those using random allocation (Schultz *et al.* 1995), but this has been challenged by a recent review that found the direction and size of any discrepancy was unpredictable (Britton *et al.* 1998).

Sometimes findings from observational studies are in direct contradiction to trial results. For example, there was evidence from many non-randomized studies that using hormone replacement therapy halves the risk of coronary heart disease (Stampfer and Colditz 1991). However, the pooled results from three randomized trials, did not show this apparent cardioprotective effect of hormone therapy (Beral *et al.* 2002). In this case, it is likely that the results from the non-randomized studies are erroneous because of residual confounding. That is, women who take hormone replacement therapy smoke less, are wealthier and take more exercise than women who do not use hormone replacement therapy. This example serves as a reminder of how we need to be cautious when interpreting the results of observational studies in health promotion.

Choosing an appropriate study design

When conducting research, particularly within the field of health promotion evaluation, the choice of whether to use a randomized or non-randomized strategy will be dictated in part by practicalities. Box 2 illustrates the basic questions to be addressed. Once a method of evaluation has been chosen, the work is only just beginning. The challenge is to design and carry out the most reliable and valid study possible. To help with the design stage, it is important to consider a number of questions, detailed in Box 2.

Box 2 Questions to ask when designing a research study

All study designs:

1. Is your study group representative of the wider population of interest?

2. Is your sample size large enough to detect an intervention effect? (Consult a statistician.)

Box 2 Questions to ask when designing a research study (Contd.)

3. How will you deal with people who do not comply with the study protocol or who are lost at follow-up?

4. Will useful evidence come from a qualitative evaluation conducted alongside the quantitative evaluation?

If a randomized controlled trial has been chosen, think about these questions:

1. What is the most efficient unit of randomizsation (individual or cluster)?

2. Is it possible to blind the trial participants to the allocation of the intervention and control?

3. Is it possible to blind the people measuring the outcome to the allocation of the intervention and control?

4. At what stage of the study will randomization occur?

If a non-randomized controlled trial has been chose, think about these questions:

1. Are the intervention and control groups similar for known confounders?

2. Can known confounders be measured at baseline and adjusted for in the analyses?

If a study with no current comparison group is chosen, think about these questions:

1. Are there any identifiable time trends (apart from the planned intervention) which are likely to distort the results? Can these be measured and adjusted for?

2. Is it possible to identify a sample (of individuals or communities) that can be studied at baseline and then at points during and after the intervention?

3. If not, how will the expected change in the population be measured?

Key points

♦ Well-conducted randomized controlled trials are a valid and important way of evaluating health promotion interventions.

♦ Randomized controlled trials are not always appropriate or possible and other forms of evaluation must be used.

♦ Randomized controlled trials are useful for measuring the effects of interventions but not for explaining why these effects occur.

References

Beral, V., Banks, F., and Reeves, G. (2002) Evidence from randomized trials on the long-term effects of hormone replacement therapy. *Lancet*, **360**, 942–944.

Britton, A. R., McKee, M., Black, N., McPherson, K., Sanderson, C., and Bain, C. (1999) Threats to applicability of randomized trials: exclusions and selective participants. *Journal of Health Services Research and Policy*, 4 (2), 112–121.

Britton, A. R., McKee, M., Black, N., McPherson, K., Sanderson, C., and Bain, C. (1998) Choosing between randomized and non-randomized studies. A systematic review. *Health Technology Assessment*, 2 (13), 1–124.

Buck, C., Llopis, A., Najera, E., and Terris, M. (1988) *The Challenge of Epidemiology: issues and selected readings*. Pan American Health Organizations, Washington, DC.

Chalmers, I. and Altman, D. G. (1995) *Systematic Reviews*. BMJ Publishing Group, London.

Hardwick, J. L., Teasdale, J., and Bloodworth, G. (1982) Caries increments over 4 years in children aged 12 at the start of the water fluoridation. *British Dental Journal*, **153**, 73–78.

John, J. H. and Ziebland, S. (2004) A comparison of anticipated and experienced barriers to eating more fruit and vegetables: A qualitative study. *Health Education Research*, 19, 165–74.

King, A. C., Haskell, W. L., Taylor, B., Kraemer, H. C., and DeBusk, R. F. (1991) Group – vs home-based exercise training in healthy older men and women. *Journal of the American Medical Association*, **266**, 1535–1542.

Medical Research Council (2000) A framework for the development and evaluation of RCTs for complex interventions to improve health. Available at http://www.mrc.ac.uk/prn/pdf-mrc_cpr.pdf

McPherson, K., Britton, A. R., and Wennberg, J. E. (1997). Are randomized controlled trials controlled? Patient preferences and unblind trials. *Journal of the Royal College of Medicine*, **90**, 652–656.

Nelson, K. E., Celentano, D. D., Eiumtrakol, S. *et al.* (1996) Changes in sexual behaviour and a decline in HIV infection among young men in Thailand. *New England Journal of Medicine*, **335**, 297–303.

Rice, V. H. and Stead, L. F. (2003) Nursing interventions for smoking cessation (Cochrane Review). In *The Cochrane Library*, Issue 4. Chichester, UK, John Wiley & Sons Ltd.

Schultz, K. F., Chalmers, I., Hayes, R. J., and Altmann, D. G. (1995) Empirical evidence of bias. Dimensions of methodological quality associated with estimates of treatment effects in controlled trials. *Journal of the American Medical Association*, **273** (5), 408–412.

Speller, V., Learmonth, A., and Harrison, D. (1997) The search for evidence of effective health promotion. *British Medical Journal*, **315**, 361–363.

Stampfer, M. J. and Colditz, G. A., (1991) Estrogen replacement therapy and coronary heart disease: a quantitative assessment of the epidemiologic evidence. *Preventive Medicine*, 2047–2063.

Stephenson, J. and Imrie, J. (1998) Why do we need randomized controlled trials to assess behavioural interventions? *British Medical Journal*, **316**, 611–613.

Chapter 6

Applying process evaluation
Learning from two research projects

Stephen Platt, Wendy Gnich,
David Rankin, Deborah Ritchie,
Julie Truman and Kathryn
Backett-Milburn

Impact and outcome evaluation, that is, establishing evidence of 'what works', are necessary, but not sufficient, components of research on the effectiveness of health promotion practice. An understanding of *how* and *why* an intervention has achieved, or failed to achieve, its objectives is also needed, and it is this that is the concern of process evaluation. Most commentators would agree with the statement by Ross *et al.* (2004 p. 177) that 'it is generally not advisable to conduct an impact evaluation without including at least a minimal process evaluation'.

This chapter introduces the purposes, focus and methods of process evaluation and explores some issues in the application of process evaluation using examples from two research projects. These issues are:

- The boundary between formative and process evaluation;
- The impact of ongoing change during the implementation of an intervention;
- The development of relationships at fieldwork sites;
- Tailoring methods to accommodate diversity; and
- Ensuring confidentiality.

What is process evaluation?

Process evaluation focuses on all aspects of delivery of an intervention, and this is why it is alternatively labelled implementation evaluation. These aspects include not only the implementation activities, but also the local context or environment and other developmental stages of the implementation process. Key components of process evaluation are listed in Table 6.1. A range of methods, both qualitative and quantitative, may be employed to collect relevant data from different stakeholder groups.

Process evaluation should be distinguished from formative evaluation, which involves a continuing exchange between research and intervention 'voices' (see also Chapter 11 for a discussion of the stages of the evaluation process). Most useful when an intervention is at an early stage, formative evaluation

> establishes the feedback mechanisms which directly affect the elements of an intervention and incorporates those processes which determine the feasibility and practicality of ideas suggested within earlier, developmental work. Formative evaluation is therefore concerned to operationalize intervention ideas and provide the research base for subsequent process and evaluations.
>
> (Flowers *et al.* 2000 p. 106)

Table 6.1 Key components of process evaluation*

Component	Definition
Context	The wider social, cultural, political and economic environment in which the intervention is embedded
Reach	Awareness and uptake of the intervention outputs by the target population
Dose delivered	The 'amount' of intervention provided by the intervention team
Dose received	The extent of engagement with the intervention shown by the target population
Fidelity	The extent to which the intervention was delivered as planned

*Adapted from Linnan and Steckler (2002: 12)

Purposes of process evaluation

Process evaluation is central to the evaluation of health promotion interventions because it serves three major purposes:

1 Describing and understanding implementation

Health promotion interventions, particularly those inspired by a community development approach, work to a loose plan and evolve in accordance with changes in both internal dynamics and external context. The interventions themselves will almost certainly be complex, and there is unlikely to be a detailed set of instructions relating to the delivery of every element. A primary concern of the researcher is, therefore, to capture *what* types of activities are being delivered, *how* they are being delivered, *why* they are being delivered, and to *whom* they are being delivered. This task is difficult. For instance, reliable methods will be required to assess the quality as well as the quantity of implementation activities, including clients' perceptions of value, cultural appropriateness and impact. The rationale for the selection of activities should be explored, as should the characteristics of clients, including the *fit* with the target group for whom the intervention was intended. *Fidelity*, that is, whether the project was implemented as intended, should be considered if there is a blueprint for the project.

2 Accounting for success (or failure)

Process evaluation helps to account for the outcome of an intervention, whether or not the intervention was effective. In the case of a successful outcome, it is important to be able to identify the components of a programme that have made a significant contribution to the overall effect, as distinct from those activities which may have had neutral or even negative consequences. More commonly, evidence of effectiveness may be confined to subgroups within the client population, and process evaluation should provide some explanation for this pattern of findings. Where there has been an unsuccessful outcome process evaluation has a role to play in accounting for the finding. Possible explanations for the lack of success that could be explored include:

- Inadequate theoretical model underpinning the intervention;
- Lack of connectedness between theoretical rationale and planned activities;
- Imperfect or incomplete implementation of the intervention;
- Change in, or failure to take account of, the context in which intervention is embedded;
- Poor quality of management or leadership.

3 Enhancing best health promotion practice

The findings of process evaluation should contribute towards the improvement of professional practice via three dissemination mechanisms. First, within the health promotion organization that has undertaken the intervention, the process evaluation can support the development of learning and improved performance. Second, findings reported to the key stakeholders can enhance mutual understanding of the barriers to, and facilitators of, intended intervention outcomes. Third, in the wider health promotion profession the process evaluation builds the knowledge base, providing evidence about interventions that should be pursued, with or without modification, or avoided.

Focus of process evaluation

The central concern of process evaluation is to understand the core activities that constitute a health promotion intervention. However, there are a number of developmental stages (described below) which may also be involved in the delivery of an intervention, and which should be evaluated. The various stages typically occur in a cyclical or overlapping, rather than linear, fashion, and each stage poses its own data collection challenges. The wider social, political, cultural and economic context should also be explored, since this has the potential to facilitate or hinder the achievement of the intervention's objectives.

Mapping

This is activity undertaken as part of a needs assessment. The aim is to gather factual and attitudinal data from intervention stakeholders and other sources to inform the development of the intervention.

Engagement

This is activity aimed at involving stakeholders, establishing their commitment, and agreeing their roles and remit. It will be important for the researcher carrying out a process evaluation to explore the understandings, perceptions and attitudes of these stakeholders.

Planning

This involves the setting and reshaping of the objectives of the intervention, as well as agreeing who is responsible and who will take the lead for specific objectives or tasks.

Implementation

This is the activity related to carrying out the intervention and includes the design and management of the intervention; provision of services, facilities and resources available; and contacts with clients.

Dissemination

Dissemination includes any activity designed to report findings to stakeholder groups. The researcher carrying out a process evaluation should supplement documentary evidence of dissemination with observation of workshops, seminars and other meetings at which verbal feedback is given (see also Chapter 12 for a discussion of evaluating dissemination of findings).

Evaluation

This is the formative and/or summative evaluation undertaken by the intervention team of individual activities that are part of the intervention.

Sustainability

To ensure the sustainability of an intervention there will be activity aimed at the continuation of the intervention by other players and the integration of intervention activities into existing structures. Exploration of the understandings and perceptions of intervention team members is not sufficient for a process evaluation in this area; the involvement of partner organizations and other stakeholders will also be necessary.

Methods of process evaluation

Given the broad scope of process evaluation, reliance on a single research method or set of methods should be avoided. Process evaluation does not rely on qualitative methods alone. Some of the monitoring activity at the heart of process evaluation, such as counting how many clients are using the service or facility, or measuring the level of client satisfaction with services, or exploring programme reach (see Table 6.1), can be most efficiently captured through the use of quantitative survey methodology. Other core evaluation questions, such as the extent to which the intervention is well organized, or the adequacy of resources or facilities, or the quality of partnership working, are best approached through the use of qualitative methods, including individual semi-structured and unstructured interviews, focus group discussions, participant observation, and documentary and textual analysis.

Example: Evaluation of Breathing Space

Breathing Space was a health promotion initiative, based on community development principles, that aimed to change the cultural climate towards smoking in a low income suburban area of Edinburgh in Scotland. Although intervention activity focused on

Example: Evaluation of Breathing Space *(Contd.)*

four main health promotion settings (community, primary care, young people [including school] and workplace), Breathing Space sought to bridge these settings and to create a health promoting environment across the wider community. There was a commitment to partnership working and multidisciplinary collaborations, and a team with representatives from each of three partner organizations (the local urban regeneration partnership, the local voluntary health agency and the local Health Board) oversaw the project. This alliance aimed to support subgroups (comprising intervention team and lay and professional community representatives) whose remit was to take forward the project objectives in each setting. In keeping with the project's community development ethos it was envisaged that professional or lay community members with no direct involvement in these formal groups would also be involved in programme activities.

The Department of Health (England) funded an evaluation of Breathing Space. In addition to an outcome evaluation using a quasi-experimental design, a comprehensive process evaluation, using a range of qualitative methods, focused on the design, development, scope, intended purpose and implementation of the programme. Two fundamental issues arose that have wider relevance for the evaluation of health promotion initiatives. The issues are, first, the decision as to whether to undertake formative feedback of process findings, and, second, the impact of ongoing change in the course of project implementation.

The utility of a formative approach?

Although there is a general consensus that a programme will be strengthened as a result of formative evaluation, there is little empirical evidence demonstrating the effects of formative evaluation on programme outcomes (Brown and Kiernan 2001).

Because Breathing Space aspired to the principles of community development, it might be expected that the findings of the process evaluation would be fed back to those involved in the intervention.

Example: Evaluation of Breathing Space (Contd.)

However, the incorporation of formative evaluation was incompatible with the use of a quasi-experimental design to assess outcome. This was because the two approaches emanate from different research paradigms (naturalistic and positivistic). The positivistic approach demands rigorous adherence to objectivity and independence of the researcher, whereas a naturalist approach celebrates the subjective understandings of research participants and the role of the researcher in the research/intervention process. Dehar *et al.* (1993) comment that formative evaluation contrasts with 'traditional conceptions of the evaluator as a neutral, detached observer'(p. 213).

In addition to this theoretical consideration, there were several likely practical consequences of using a formative approach. First, the evaluation team was aware that reporting findings could have a negative impact on the morale of implementers and the course of implementation. Where there is internal discord and disagreement during the course of implementation, as was the case in Breathing Space, feedback may exacerbate already strained relationships.

Second, formative evaluation has implications for the relationship between researchers and participants and therefore for the quality of the data. For example, because evaluators may be perceived as experts on community interventions, aspects of programme feedback may assume particular importance or exert undue influence. The potential for such an effect will be heightened when, as in Breathing Space, implementers are uncertain about how to achieve programme objectives while upholding underlying principles.

Third, it is possible that feedback from the research team might conflict with the 'natural' development of the programme to the detriment of its community capacity-building aims, although it is arguable that conflict is a necessary component of that process. How feedback is interpreted and acted upon will depend very much on the status of the recipient group (e.g. workers or managers), their cultural norms and their level of mutual support. Where a multi-agency partnership exists, as in Breathing Space, the response to

Example: Evaluation of Breathing Space *(Contd.)*

feedback will also depend on inter-organizational support. Both the content and process of feedback may affect participants' perceptions of, and willingness to engage with, the research team.

Working with change: a developmental process

A second issue arose because of the multiple ways in which the initiative and its wider context changed over the course of the evaluation. Long-term community development programmes such as Breathing Space tend to evolve over the implementation period.

In order to plan and implement a programme evaluation, evaluators prefer to know what the programme is, what it will comprise, and what its objectives are. Because the objectives, activities and structures of Breathing Space were developed and agreed by a lengthy process of community consultation they were not clear at the outset. Answering these key questions was therefore a central task of the process evaluation. Moreover, the answers were not fixed but required constant revisiting as objectives, activities and structures were re-shaped throughout the implementation period. This 'question answering' or documentation process was a necessary prerequisite to the development of a comprehensive process evaluation method, since it was imperative to identify which stakeholders would be participating in which meetings and implementing which activities before the most suitable evaluation methods could be identified. Inevitably, not all stakeholders with a central role in the initiation of the programme were actively involved throughout its life, while others who did not envisage themselves as having a role at the outset became increasingly involved. Thus, process evaluation methods were required which would both capture the fluid nature of the intervention and respond to it.

Despite anticipating the evolutionary developmental process that characterized Breathing Space, the extent of change was underestimated. The process evaluation documented numerous

Example: Evaluation of Breathing Space (Contd.)

changes that were neither intended nor a direct result of the community development approach. In particular, Breathing Space was adversely affected by a large number of staff changes throughout its life. Restructuring in all three of the programme's main partner organizations exacerbated this turnover. The effects of these changes had major implications for the project and they also impacted on the research process. The ability to gather accurate and detailed process evaluation data was reliant on stakeholders' goodwill and commitment to evaluation. This was in turn determined by participants' understandings of the role and purpose of the evaluation. Thus, frequent staff changes necessitated ongoing explanation of the research process, negotiation of participant roles and the re-establishment of trusting relationships between the evaluation team and new or replacement personnel.

A reduction in the funding available from other sources for tobacco and wider health promotion work during the programme period and contextual changes occurring elsewhere had important implications for the interpretation of evaluation outcomes. Process monitoring in both intervention and control communities highlighted unexpected factors that had the potential to alter the 'net dose' of activity delivered in the intervention area. New process methods were incorporated in response to these changes in order to account for possible effects on the research design. For example, following the release of the Smoking Kills White Paper (Secretary of State for Health 1998) smoking cessation activity organized by Local Health Care Co-operatives was monitored. Similarly, once nicotine replacement therapy and Buproprion ('Zyban') were made available on prescription, area-based prescribing data were requested from the local health board. A full time research fellow worked as evaluator of the programme throughout its duration and this enabled changes to be tracked and logged. The evaluator was in frequent contact with all aspects of the programme's operation. This was vital to ensure that the process methods remained flexible to both anticipated and unanticipated change.

Example: Evaluation of the Healthy Living Centre programme in Scotland

Healthy Living Centres (HLCs) are expected to promote good health in its broadest sense, particularly focusing upon the most disadvantaged in society, and to reduce health inequalities. Users and local communities are encouraged to play an active role in HLC design and delivery to ensure that the focus is on the needs of communities. Other intermediate outcomes of the programme include promoting social inclusion, building partnership work between sectors and agencies, and ensuring project sustainability.

The Scottish Executive Health Department has commissioned an evaluation of the Healthy Living Centres programme in Scotland during 2002–04. The objectives of the study are:

1. To undertake an intensive evaluation of a sample of HLC projects in terms of:
   - the linkages between activities,
   - the mechanisms for effecting change in health and health-related behaviour,
   - the local context and actual outcomes;

2. To provide the Scottish Executive with detailed evidence about the contribution of the HLC programme to key strategic aims, such as the reduction of health inequalities, the promotion of partnership working for health, and the encouragement of community participation;

3. To assist HLCs and their partners to learn from the experience; and

4. To be of relevance to other policy initiatives with a direct or indirect health focus.

The challenge of a multi-site process evaluation is to combine the gathering of comparable data across all HLCs with obtaining in-depth illuminative data that reflect each site's unique history and implementation. A sample of six HLCs has been selected

Example: Evaluation of the Healthy Living Centre programme in Scotland (Contd.)

which reflects the range of interests, anticipated health outcomes and geographical locations of projects within Scotland. A case-study design, incorporating two periods of intensive fieldwork one year apart, permits an in-depth investigation of processes within each HLC. During planning of fieldwork the research team has taken into account the relationship required between evaluators and participants. As a result of the disparate nature of the sample, the evaluation has been required to accommodate each site's unique configuration, partner alliances, target groups, geographical coverage and intended health outcomes.

Consideration was given to ethical issues and the political process of negotiation (Punch 1998), so that the research team could make successful initial contact and maintain access with each HLC, recognizing their unique developmental and operational elements. Ethical concerns primarily comprised issues of harm, consent, privacy and confidentiality of data (Punch 1998). Political considerations had to take into account personal relations, cultures of universities, cultures of organizations examined, policies of funding bodies and also those of central government (Bell and Newby 1977, Hammond 1964). Accommodating the variations within each HLC affected how the process evaluation proceeded.

Negotiating and ensuring continued access to people and places

A series of workshops, to which selected HLCs were invited, offered opportunities to discuss the aims and objectives of the evaluation and potential methods that might be used. The workshops also enabled project coordinators and selected staff to elucidate the connections between their project's aims, outputs, short-term and longer term outcomes using an adapted version of the basic logic model (W. K. Kellogg Foundation 2001). Six HLCs

Example: Evaluation of the Healthy Living Centre programme in Scotland (Contd.)

were invited to participate in the evaluation and all accepted. During an initial visit to each site by a junior and senior member of the research team, future fieldwork plans were developed, and work settings and local contexts were explored.

The researcher identified and established a relationship with a project gatekeeper, as this has been found to be crucial to gain access to social research sites (Argyris 1969). The gatekeeper was in most instances the project coordinator and one of the people who had attended the workshop, although on one occasion the lead partner of an HLC had an overseeing role and acted as the gatekeeper. Further negotiations then took place between the researcher and gatekeeper to obtain background documentation such as business plans, minutes of meetings and relevant reports in advance of going into the field. Identifying key individuals to participate in the evaluation involved discussion with the gatekeepers to determine which stakeholders had strategic or operational knowledge about the HLC. This gave gatekeepers an influence over the evaluation, as they may have selected favoured stakeholders or partners to participate. On several occasions gatekeepers also helped to smooth the path when approaching hard-to-reach target users during fieldwork, as many vulnerable and sensitive groups were involved. Good long-term working relationships were important: the gatekeepers acted as the principal contact between periods of fieldwork, ensuring prolonged access to the site and providing opportunities to follow-up how work was progressing.

The emphasis placed on developing and maintaining relationships with HLCs and key individuals assisted the evaluation in a variety of ways. First, the degree of openness between researchers and researched seems to have broken down some of the mystery and anxiety surrounding the evaluation process. Second, this openness created a welcoming environment for evaluators and in many instances led to the divulging of information that had not

Example: Evaluation of the Healthy Living Centre programme in Scotland (Contd.)

originally been requested. Finally, there was early evidence of a perceived lack of opportunity for organizations participating in the HLC programme to network with each other. Comments received about the evaluation workshops indicated that these had been seen as a useful mechanism for meeting other HLC coordinators and staff.

Using and tailoring methods – keeping everyone happy

The intensive approach adopted during the Scottish HLC evaluation was designed to generate data that could also be relevant to a linked UK-wide evaluation of the HLC programme. The principal methods used were semi-structured interviews (face-to-face and group), observation of a range of settings and activities, and documentary analysis. The development of the organization and the personnel structure of each HLC were important considerations when devising the instruments. Across and sometimes within the participating HLCs there were variations in start-up times, structures of management, deployment of staff, types and numbers of partner organizations, use of volunteers, levels of community involvement and user groups.

Instruments were customized for each site following the collection and assimilation of information from background documentation.

Each HLC provided a different quantity of information, the quality of which often only became apparent when interviews were conducted. In many instances changes or expansion had occurred in both the structure and level of operation of the HLC since bid documents and business plans had been compiled. Consequently the researcher had to adjust and remain responsive to the information divulged by participants during fieldwork.

Example: Evaluation of the Healthy Living Centre programme in Scotland *(Contd.)*

Instruments for user groups also had to be refined depending on the characteristics of target interviewees, who came from a wide spectrum of society including, for instance, young homeless people, older housebound groups, people experiencing mental health problems and entire communities within a geographical location.

Doing no harm – trying to ensure confidentiality

Informed consent was sought from all participants, whenever possible (e.g. before formal interviews); however, in some instances, such as during observations at school events where an HLC was providing activities, this was not possible. It was important to make participants aware that the evaluation team sought to gather data from both formal and informal contacts and not only during taped interviews. In accordance with the research team's commitment to ensuring the anonymity of respondents and the confidentiality of data obtained, reporting of contentious issues of a personal nature was handled with extreme sensitivity when providing HLCs with interim feedback.

Despite this stance the research team experienced several dilemmas when faced with frank stakeholder accounts that, if made public, had the potential to cause harm to other participants. Even sharing information within the research team was problematic; a coding system had to be developed to safeguard anonymity and confidentiality when data were transferred electronically or transported as hard copy. It remains a challenge for any research team to reach consensus as to what information a researcher can, or should, divulge to other members of the team or to a wider audience, while seeking to do no harm to research participants or to the integrity of the evaluation.

Conclusion

Increasing emphasis is being placed on the importance of evidence and knowledge about what works as a basis for the development and implementation of health promotion practice. Where evidence is lacking or not generalizable to specific contexts, it is expected that the effectiveness of an intervention will be assessed through primary empirical research. It is now widely accepted that such an assessment must include a rigorous and appropriate evaluation of process. The importance of comprehensive process evaluation to document the history of interventions and enable fuller understanding of their outcomes cannot be overemphasized. This chapter has sought to describe the characteristics, purposes, focus and methods of process evaluation and, using examples from two research projects in which the authors have been involved, to explore several issues in the application of process evaluation. Its goal has been to persuade readers of the value of incorporating an assessment of process into the evaluation research programme, while recognizing the challenges that face the research team aspiring to undertake high quality work in this area.

Key points

- Process evaluation provides a description of all aspects of the implementation of a health promotion intervention.

- Understanding of *how* and *why* an intervention has achieved, or failed to achieve, its objectives is the central concern of process evaluation.

- Process evaluation requires the rigorous application of both quantitative and qualitative methods.

- Process evaluation methods must be tailored to the particular characteristics of the intervention being evaluated.

- The challenge of establishing good working relationships at fieldwork sites and tailoring methods to accommodate diversity should not be underestimated.

References

Argyris, C. (1969) Diagnosing defences against the outsider. In G. J. McCall and J. L. Simmons (eds) *Issues in Participant Observation*. Addison-Wesley, Reading, MA.

Bell, C. and Newby, H. (eds) (1977) *Doing Sociological Research*. Allen & Unwin, London.

Brown, J. L. and Kiernan, N. E. (2001) Assessing the subsequent effect of a formative evaluation on a program. *Evaluation and Program Planning*, 24 (2), 129–143.

Dehar, M., Casswell, S., and Duignan, P. (1993) Formative and process evaluation of health promotion and disease prevention programs. *Evaluation Review*, 17 (2), 204–220.

Flowers, P., Frankis, J., and Hart, G. (2000) Evidence and the evaluation of a community-level intervention. Researching the Gay Men's Task Force initiative. In J. Watson and S. Platt (eds) *Researching Health Promotion*. Routledge, London.

Hammond, P. (ed.) (1964) *Sociologists at Work*. Basic Books, New York.

Linnan, L. and Steckler, A. (2002) Process evaluation for public health interventions and research: an overview. In A. Steckler and L. Linnan (eds) *Process Evaluation for Public Health Interventions and Research*. Jossey-Bass, San Francisco, CA.

Punch, M. (1998) Politics and ethics in qualitative research. In N. K. Denzin and Y. S. Lincoln (eds) *The Landscape of Qualitative Research: Theories and Issues*. Sage, London.

Ross, P. H., Lipsey M. W., and Freeman, H. E. (2004) *Evaluation. A Systematic Approach*, 7th edn. Sage, Thousand Oaks, CA.

Secretary of State for Health (1998) *Smoking Kills. A White Paper on Tobacco* (Cm 4177). The Stationery Office, London.

W. K. Kellogg Foundation (2001) Using logic models to bring together planning, evaluation, and action. Logic model development guide. <http://www.wkkf.org/Pubs/Tools/Evaluation/Pub3669.pdf>

Part III

Evaluation in practice

Chapter 7

Evaluating social marketing interventions

Steven Chapman

A process, perspective and strategy of health promotion

Social marketing is a process for designing and modifying health promotion interventions. Commercial marketers characterize their offerings to customers in terms of the 'marketing mix' – a combination of the 4Ps of product, price, place and promotion. For example, automobile manufacturers design and offer cars that are big or small, expensive or cheap, widely or exclusively available, or sporty or traditional in look depending on the perceptions of self interest of a given population and the offerings of competing manufacturers or suppliers of transportation. Similarly, social marketing characterizes and manages health promotion interventions in terms of the 4Ps.

Social marketing broadly defines products as a bundle of benefits that range from an actual product or service, such as a condom in an HIV/AIDS campaign, to ideas related to a desired behaviour, such as safer sex, and the associated perceived benefits of that behaviour, such as the peace of mind that comes from knowing that one is likely to remain HIV negative (Kotler, Roberto and Lee 2002). Social marketing seeks to enhance this 'product' in a manner that makes it more appealing to populations than competing products, services, and ideas, for example not using a condom or not knowing one's HIV status. Price is seen as the monetary and perceived non-monetary costs associated with adopting the behaviour. Social marketers seek to minimize those costs such that the behaviour is 'easy' (Andreasen 2002b). Place is either physical or the perceived potential access to the product or service or, more broadly, to where the behaviour is performed, such as the home, workplace, school, health centre, store, bar, or community. Social marketing generally seeks to maximize potential access in terms of where the behaviour is performed and to do so cost-effectively. Promotion is persuasive communication, both mass media and interpersonal, regarding the product, service, or idea, and the price at which and place where it can be accessed.

The social marketing process is therefore a series of steps characterized by when and how the social marketer interacts with the population of interest to define, deliver and modify the 4Ps. The first step is a systematic effort to understand the population's perceived self-interest in the behaviour or set of behaviours whose change would lead to an improvement in health status and quality of life. Next, social marketers iteratively develop the 4Ps based on population preferences and reactions first to concepts and then to a more defined social marketing intervention. The social marketing intervention is then conducted, with mechanisms put in place to monitor and evaluate changes in behaviour, perceptions, and potential access. Lastly, one or more of the 4Ps is modified as behaviour, perceptions and potential access change over time.

Social marketing is a perspective on health promotion, not a theory (Glanz, Rimer and Lewis 2002, Valente 2002). Within interventions planned under any health behaviour theory, such as the Health Belief Model or Social Cognitive Theory, social marketing applies concepts from commercial marketing and exchange theory, such as appealing to self interest and addressing competition, to enable people to respond to interventions. Commercial marketers have learned that people are motivated to buy cars, subscribe to mobile phone plans or eat organically-grown foods when they perceive these products, services or ideas to be in their self interest and superior to competing offers. People list a range of self-interests in choosing, for example, a car to buy, from the more rational, such as the need for transportation, to the more emotional and sensational, such as a desire to increase their social status and sex appeal. These perceived self interests can be shaped by marketing efforts into strong preferences for specific brands and a willingness to spend money and effort and sacrifice other opportunities to buy and own them. Social marketing uses these concepts in health promotion interventions to identify and appeal to self interests both rational, such as the benefit of

preserving or improving one's own health, and emotional and sensational, such as the promise of fresh breath and self-confidence while kiss-
ing, offered as a benefit of stopping smoking (Berman 2003). Social
marketing encourages health promoters to design interventions to com-
pete with those things that people genuinely enjoy or benefit from in the
current behaviour, such as the feeling of belonging when smoking with
a group of friends who also smoke. Social marketers believe that people
will voluntarily exchange these perceived benefits for others that are
associated with individually or socially-beneficial behaviours, but only if
the marketer designs and delivers products, services or ideas that are
superior to the benefits being given up. This voluntary exchange marks
the measure of success for social marketing, and distinguishes it in organizational and ethical terms from commercial marketing (Smith 2001).

Social marketing is a behaviour change strategy increasingly applied
to health and other social issues (Rothschild 1999). It was first suggested
in the 1950s in a response to the question 'Why can't you sell brother-
hood like soap?' (Weibe 1951–1952). Family planning programmes
in developing countries adopted social marketing in the 1960s and
1970s by marketing contraceptives through private sector channels at
subsidized prices (Harvey 1999). In the 1980s, social marketing grew
increasingly popular through evidence of its effectiveness in heart
health and other health promotion programmes and efforts to define its
principles and processes more precisely (Lefebvre and Rochlin 1996). In
the 1990s, social marketing applications expanded steadily and rapidly
to HIV/AIDS and maternal and child health interventions in developing
countries, and to a range of health, safety, environmental and
community mobilization interventions in the developed world (Kotler,
Roberto and Lee 2002, Hastings and Haywood 1991). Today, social
marketing for health promotion provides an alternative to purely
educationally-based strategies that are unable to increase potential access
to products and services, or purely regulatory-based strategies that
use non-voluntary approaches to induce behaviour changes.

The role of evaluation in social marketing

Evaluation in social marketing has been described as an inherently
practical exercise aimed at determining how to improve interventions (Balch and Sutton 1997). Evaluations are most useful if they

are integrated into programmes in an interactive, iterative, and continuous system. Evaluation systems should be capable of repeatedly answering three questions relevant to the social marketing decision maker, namely What should we do (segmentation and 4P development)? How are we doing (monitoring)? And How did we do (evaluation)?

The aim of a social marketing evaluation system is characterized differently in health and purely social marketing terms. In health terms, continuous evaluation permits evidence-based decision-making. In social marketing terms, such a system allows the marketer to be continuously customer driven or focused (Andreasen 2002b). Balch and Sutton (1997) specify the required characteristics of such a system as being able to provide relevant, accurate, timely, and cost-effective feedforward and feedback on plans, target segments, behaviour change processes and impact for social marketers and their stakeholders.

The challenge of building such evaluation systems for both commercial and social marketing led to the development of the backward research methodology (Andreasen 2002a). The name comes from the method's starting point, the analytical tables or structure of the research report itself, which are drafted as the first step of the research process, rather than the last. Backward research is essentially the adaptation of the social marketing process to the process of designing and delivering an evaluation. To apply the backward research process, the social marketing evaluator must have the resources, skills, and motivation to play the role of a key social marketing team member (Balch and Sutton 1997). Social marketing evaluation itself can then be held accountable to social marketers and other stakeholders in terms of the extent to which its findings result in evidence-based decision-making and improved intervention performance.

PERForM: A performance framework for social marketing

The primary issue in social marketing evaluation, just as in any health promotion evaluation, is the causal association between exposure to the social marketing intervention and changes in the theoretically derived determinants of behaviour, behaviour change, and health status. Yet, because the theoretically derived determinants of behaviour that social marketing can affect include expanding potential access to products, services and ideas, a social marketing intervention must also be evaluated in terms of its role within the health system itself. Health systems evaluation considers, in addition to effectiveness, other measures of performance evaluation such as cost-effectiveness, equity, coverage, quality, access, and interactions with other determinants of health status. Figure 7.1 depicts PERForM (a PERformance Framework for social Marketing used by Population Services International). The framework is based on the Behavioural Model of Health Services Use (Andersen 1995).

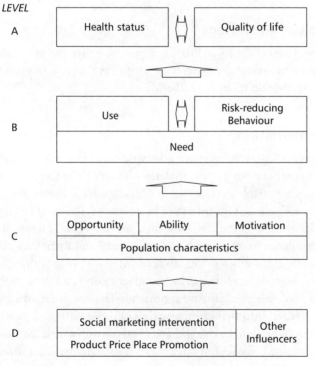

Fig. 7.1 PERForM

PERForM has four levels, A to D. Level A consists of the goal of social marketing for health promotion – improved health status or, for interventions relating to coping with sickness and disability, quality of life. Level B consists of the objectives of health promotion programmes, stated as product or service use on the left side and/or other risk-reducing behaviours that do not involve the use of a product or service on the right side. The adoption or maintenance of these behaviours in the presence of a given need or vulnerability is causally antecedent to improving or maintaining health and/or quality of life. Level C consists of the determinants of behaviour summarized in terms of opportunity, ability and motivation, given a set of population characteristics, that respond to Level D, the social marketing intervention or other influences of health, including health education, regulation, or other trends and impulses present in society.

Evaluation strategy

At each step of the social marketing process, either qualitative and or quantitative research strategies are used to evaluate social marketing interventions in terms of PERForM.

Segmentation

Social marketers first *segment* otherwise heterogeneous populations into homogenous groups that are *identifiable* in terms of easily measured variables, *substantial* in size, *accessible* to the intervention, *stable* long enough for the 4Ps to be developed, delivered and evaluated, *responsive* to the marketing mix, and *actionable* in terms of giving guidance to 4P decision-making (Wedel and Kamakura 2000). The population is a priori divided into two groups, those with a health need (including a risk or vulnerability) and those without such need, using quantitative approaches. Those with a need are then subdivided into two groups again (1) those with a need whose behaviour needs to be changed and (2) those with a need that already perform the behaviour of interest. Those without need are hereafter no longer of interest.

Next, the social marketer compares *post hoc* the two remaining groups in terms of Level C constructs that are theoretically responsive to the social marketing interventions. The aim is to identify significant differences between the two groups in terms of opportunity, ability and motivation. These constructs are operationalized into questions, first through qualitative research strategies that define theoretically identified population perceptions, and then into multi-item scales using quantitative approaches for scale validation.

Opportunity

This refers to community and service factors that promote or inhibit the behaviour of interest (Rothschild 1999). Opportunity constructs are derived from diffusion of innovation theory, health promotion and quality of care research and include measures of perceived access to products, services and ideas, perceived quality of care, and the appeal of the specific attributes of currently available or proposed products and services in terms of the 4Ps.

Ability

This refers to an individual's perceived proficiency at solving problems, given the setting, opportunity and motivation (Rothschild 1999). Ability constructs can come from economics, such as measures of willingness to pay for accessing products, services or ideas, and social psychology, such as social cognitive and other theories that examine social norms and support, self-efficacy, and other interpersonal determinants of behaviour change.

Motivation

Motivation describes how a person has self-interest in changing his or her behaviour, given the opportunity and ability (Rothschild 1999). Motivational constructs that are most proximate to behaviour may include personal risk assessment, outcome expectations, or, for family planning, fertility intentions. Those that are more distal from behaviour and that may influence these proximate constructs may relate among other things to trust and caution in sexual relations, awareness of the behaviour and its benefits and costs, or emotional reactions to related past events.

Next, the social marketer determines whether correlations between behaviour, given need, and significant opportunity, ability and motivation constructs vary by population characteristics, including demographic, socio-economic, and geographic or other access-oriented variables. The result is the identification of one or more sets of opportunity, ability and motivation determinants that, if changed in the group that is currently not behaving in a health-promoting manner, would maximize the likelihood of behaviour change (Meekers and Klein 2001). Lastly, the social marketer evaluates the identified segment in terms of its substantiality and accessibility. The stability of the segment over the period of the intervention is assumed.

Environmental/market analysis

The second step of the social marketing process is to conduct an environmental and market analysis relating to the Level C opportunity construct. In contrast to the segmentation step above in which individual level characteristics and perceptions are examined and measured, here expertly defined indicators of access to products and services and the quality of care available are measured.

Strategic, intervention and marketing planning

The presence or absence of significant associations between Level C opportunity, ability and motivation constructs and Level B objectives and the results of the environmental/market analysis guide the decision whether social marketing is a useful or actionable strategy for behaviour change singularly or in combination with other educational or regulatory strategies (Rothschild 1999). Intervention goals and objectives are then set related to changes in Levels A, B, and C, given a planned 'dose' of Level D exposures. Marketing plans are developed using qualitative and quantitative strategies used to generate and pre-test Level D 4P concepts.

Monitoring and evaluation are then based on the measures of social marketing performance presented below.

Measures of social marketing performance

PERForM defines eight primary measures for evaluating social marketing performance.

Effectiveness

Effectiveness is defined as a causal association between Level D exposures and changes at Level C (opportunity, ability and motivation), Level B (behaviour) and or Level A (health status and or quality of life), given need, and adjusting for other influencers of behaviour.

Cost-effectiveness

Cost-effectiveness is defined as the cost at Level D of producing a marginal change at Levels C, B, and A.

Substitution and halo effects

A substitution effect is a negative, unintended impact in which one behaviour is increased, but use of an equally beneficial behaviour is decreased. In HIV/AIDS programmes, for example, policy makers seek to monitor a specific type of substitution effect known as disinhibition in which potentially a campaign aimed at increasing the use of condoms may be found effective, but also results in a decrease in risk reducing behaviour such as abstinence or fidelity to one sexual partner. A halo effect is a positive, unintended impact in which efforts to increase one behaviour also results in increases in other, positive behaviours. An example might be when physical activity is effectively promoted within a heart health programme, and the same promotion also is found to be causally associated with other behavioural changes such as improved nutrition or avoidance of tobacco.

Equity

Equity in health services research is defined as the absence of a difference in the use of a health product or service or the practice of a risk reducing behaviour, given need, across socio-economic strata. Many social marketing interventions state a priori a preference for targeting populations of lower socio-economic status to reduce differences at Levels A and B by socio-economic status. Socio-economic status can be defined as income, expenditure or asset ownership, or other population characteristics such as education, sex, and residence (Andersen 1995).

Coverage

Coverage is the proportion of geographically defined areas in which the product, service or idea promoted by the social marketing intervention is available.

Quality of care

Quality of care is the proportion of geographically defined areas or service delivery points in which the product, service or idea is delivered in compliance with minimum standards.

Equity of access

Equity of access occurs when, among population segments with equal levels of need, risk or vulnerability, there is equal geographically-defined access to products, services and or ideas.

Efficiency

Efficiency is the cost-effectiveness of the social marketing intervention in settings with equity of access.

The social marketing evidence base

Evidence of the performance of social marketing for health promotion is accumulating, particularly with regard to HIV/AIDS, maternal and child health, and family planning and reproductive health interventions in developing countries and nutrition and physical activity interventions for heart health, cancer and diabetes in the developed world (Chapman and Astatke 2003, Alcalay and Bell 2000). Evidence relating to the impact of social marketing on health status is more readily available for interventions in the developed rather than in the developing world. Alcalay and Bell (2000) reported that 16 of 44 published studies (38%) examining nutrition and physical activity interventions primarily in developed countries measured clinical changes in health status. By contrast, in developing countries, only 8 of 66 studies (12%) reported impact on health status, yet the extent of that impact, particularly with regard to malaria mortality and morbidity, is remarkable (Holtz *et al.* 2002, Abdulla *et al.* 2001, Rowland *et al.* 2002, Schellenberg *et al.* 2001).

Examples: measuring impact on health status

In Tanzania, Schellenberg *et al.* (2001) found that an insecticide-treated mosquito net social marketing intervention averted 5% of deaths in children ages one month to four years. In Malawi, both rural and urban children under five who slept under insecticide-treated nets, most of which were supplied by the social marketing intervention, had significantly lower levels of anemia and parasitemia (Holtz *et al.* 2002).

Nearly all evaluations of social marketing interventions, in both developed and developing countries, report impact on behaviour change, both product and service use and the practice of risk-reducing behaviour. For example, in developing countries, interventions have been found effective in increasing the use of

condoms, oral contraceptives, insecticide-treated nets and reproductive health services. Evaluations of non-product behaviours have
found social marketing to be effective in increasing abstinence and
fidelity, and several preventive child health behaviours, including
hand washing for diarrhoeal disease prevention.

Approximately half of reported social marketing interventions in
both the developed and developing world report impact on the
determinants of behaviour in the areas of opportunity, ability and
motivation. Evidence from developing countries has increased
substantially since 2000 and shows that social marketing increases
knowledge about opportunities to use products and the source
of those products (e.g Van Rossem and Meekers 2000, Agha 2002).
It has effects on social norms and perceived self-efficacy that
are associated with the adoption of healthy behaviours. It also
increases risk perceptions and awareness of the need to adopt
preventive behaviours. Social marketing creates intentions to change
behaviour and motivation to continue that changed behaviour.

Evidence of cost-effectiveness, substitution and halo effects, equity,
coverage, quality, equity of access and efficiency is substantially less
common. These are areas where more evaluation is needed.
Nevertheless, the published evidence shows positive effects in both
developing and developed countries.

Examples: measuring cost-effectiveness

For water and sanitation programmes in the developing world,
one study reported that the cost per disability-adjusted life-year-
averted of social marketing was less than US$150, and thus under
the threshold set by the World Bank for classifying an intervention as highly cost-effective (Varley et al. 1998). In Louisiana, in
the United States, another study found that a 30% increase in
condom use averted 170 HIV infections, saved 1,909 quality-
adjusted life-years, and $33 million in care costs. Sensitivity
analysis found that a 2.7% increase in condom use would result
in the interventions being cost-effective (Bedimo et al. 2002).

Example: measuring halo and substitution effects

A family planning intervention in Honduras provides evidence of both halo and substitution effects. There, 45% of women using social marketing oral contraceptives were new users. In addition about 25% of the users had switched from the public sector – a likely halo effect or positive interaction in terms of increasing the overall efficiency of the health system since the cost of product delivery was shifted from government financing to those willing to pay at least a portion of the cost of the product. The remainder had switched from the commercial sector – a substitution effect or negative interaction since the cost of product delivery had initially been paid wholly by the client and now was partially subsidized through social marketing (Bailey, Janowitz, Solis, Machuca and Suazo 1989). The same intervention provided evidence of the equity impact of social marketing. New users of the social marketing oral contraceptive in Honduras were less educated, less likely to live in homes with electricity and had lower quality sanitation facilities than new users of commercial brands (Bailey *et al.* 1989).

Example: measuring equity

In Malawi, no significant differences between social marketing and community-based and clinic users were found in urban and rural areas of a non-governmental organization programme by socio-economic status, either when examined alone or in combination with educational status (Janowitz *et al.* 1992).

Significant gaps remain in the social marketing evidence base that exists to guide practitioners and planners in designing and evaluating interventions (Chapman and Astatke 2003). For example, in both developed and developing countries, additional evidence is needed relating to price as a potential barrier to continued use of products and services or the adoption of risk-reducing behaviours. Evidence of a dose-response relative to the intensity of the intervention and the resulting impact is currently overly focused on the relationship between promotion and ability and motivation, while the other '3Ps' of marketing and their relationship to changes in all salient measures of opportunity, ability and motivation are less well understood.

An agenda for improving the evaluation of social marketing interventions

Substantial barriers exist to filling gaps in the social marketing evidence base and improving social marketing evaluation and performance. Much more attention and investment is required to establish tracking surveys – cross-sectional, representative surveys of populations and delivery systems – to produce actionable reports of the PERForM measures. Strategic planning based on segmentation and an understanding of the roles of social marketing, education, and regulation remains uncommon. Outside of heart health, interventions and evaluations based on single behaviours remain commonplace, when arguably providing multiple, related behavioural options and segmenting on these could increase intervention cost-effectiveness. Evaluators and social marketers need to learn more about each other's capabilities and techniques in order to have evaluators become key members of social marketing programme teams, to increase the use of evidence-based decision-making in social marketing and to improve the accountability of evaluation to social marketing stakeholders.

Key points

- Social marketing is a process for designing and modifying health promotion interventions.
- Social marketing incorporates the known theories of behaviour change and then applies commercial marketing and exchange theory concepts to design and evaluate interventions.

Key points *(Contd.)*

- Evaluation in social marketing is an inherently practical exercise aimed at determining how to improve social marketing interventions.

- The PERForM framework defines the scope and measures of performance for social marketing across the steps of the social marketing process.

- Evidence of the performance of social marketing for health promotion is accumulating, yet significant gaps in the evidence base remain for measures other than effectiveness.

References

Abdulla, S., Schellenberg, J. A., Nathan, R., Mukasa, O., Marchant, T., Smith, T., Tanner, M., and Lengeler, C. (2001) Impact on malaria morbidity of a programme supplying insecticide treated nets in children aged under 2 years in Tanzania: Community cross sectional study. *British Medical Journal*, **322**, 270–273.

Agha, S. (2002) A quasi-experimental study to assess the impact of four adolescent sexual health interventions in Sub-saharan Africa. *International Family Planning Perspectives*, **28**, 67–70; 113–118.

Alcalay, R. and Bell, R. A. (2000) *Promoting Nutrition and Physical Activity through Social Marketing: Current practices and recommendations.* Center for Advanced Studies in Nutrition and Social Marketing, University of California, Davis, CA.

Andersen, R. M. (1995). Revisiting the behavioural model and access to medical care: does it matter? *Journal of Health and Social Behaviour*, **36**, 1–10.

Andreasen, A. (2002a) *Marketing Research that won't Break the Bank: A practical guide to getting the information you need*, 2nd edn, pp. 60–74. San Francisco, CA, Jossey-Bass.

Andreasen, A. (2002b) Marketing social marketing in the social change marketplace. *Journal of Public Policy and Marketing*, **21**, 3–13.

Bailey, P. E., Janowitz, B., Solis, M., Machuca, M., and Suazo, M. (1989) Consumers of oral contraceptives in a social marketing campaign in Honduras. *Studies in Family Planning*, **20**, 53–61.

Balch, G. I. and Sutton, S. M. (1997) Keep me posted: a plea for practical evaluation. In M. E. Goldberg, M. Fishbein, and S. E. Middlestadt (eds) *Social Marketing: Theoretical and Practical Perspectives.* Lawrence Erlbaum Associates, Inc., Mahwah, NJ.

Bedimo, A. L., Pinkerton, S. D., Cohen, D. A., Gray, B., and Farley, T. A. (2002) Condom distribution: a cost-utility analysis. *International Journal of STD and AIDS*, **13**, 384–392.

Berman, J. (2003) Personal communication.

Chapman, S. and Astatke, H. (2003) *The Social Marketing Evidence Base. Social Marketing Research Series.* Population Services International, Washington, DC.

Glanz, K., Rimer, B. K., and Lewis, F. M. (2002). *Health Behavior and Health Education.* Jossey-Bass, San Francisco, CA.

Harvey, P. (1999) *Let Every Child Be Wanted: How social marketing is revolutionizing family planning programs in the developing world.* Auburn House, Westport, CT.

Hastings, G. and Haywood, A. (1991) Social marketing and communication for health promotion. *Health Promotion International*, **6**, 135–145.

Holtz, T. H., Marum, L. H., Mkandala, C., Chizani, N., Roberts, J. M., Macheso, A., Parise, M. E., and Kachur, S. P. (2002) Insecticide-treated bednet use, anaemia, and malaria parasitaemia in Blantyre District, Malawi. *Tropical Medicine and International Health*, **7**, 220–230.

Janowitz, B., Suazo, M., Fried, D. B., Bratt, J. H., and Bailey, P. E. (1992) Impact of social marketing on contraceptive prevalence and cost in Honduras. *Studies in Family Planning*, **23**, 110–117.

Kotler, P., Roberto, N., and Lee, N. (2002) *Social Marketing: Improving the quality of life.* Sage Publications, Inc, Thousand Oaks, CA.

Lefebvre, R. C. and Rochlin, L. (1996) Social marketing. In K. Glanz, F. M. Lewis and B. K. Rimer (eds) *Health Behavior and Health Education: Theory, Research and Practice.* Jossey-Bass, San Francisco, CA.

Meekers, D. and Klein, M. (2001) Determinants of condom use among unmarried youth in Yaounde and Douala. *PSI Working Paper No 47.* Population Services International, Washington, DC.

Rothschild, M. (1999) Carrots, sticks, and promises: A conceptual framework for the management of public health and social issue behaviors. *Journal of Marketing*, **63**, 24–37.

Rowland, M., Webster, J., Saleh, P., Chandramohan, D., Freeman, T., Pearcy, B., Durrani, N., Rab, A., and Mohammed, N. (2002) Prevention of malaria in Afghanistan through social marketing of insecticide-treated nets: evaluation of coverage and effectiveness by cross-sectional surveys and passive surveillance. *Tropical Medicine and International Health*, **7**, 813–822.

Schellenberg, J. R., Abdulla, S., Nathan, R., Mukasa, O., Marchant, T. J., Kikumbih, N., Mushi, A. K., Mponda, H., Minja, H., Mshinda, H., Tanner, M., and Lengeler, C. (2001) Effect of large-scale social marketing of insecticide-treated nets on child survival in rural Tanzania. *Lancet*, **357**, 1241–1247.

Smith, W. A. (2001) Ethics and the social marketer: A framework for practitioners. In A. R. Andreasen (ed.) *Ethics in Social Marketing*. Georgetown University Press, Washington, DC.

Valente, T. W. (2002) *Evaluating Health Promotion Programs*. Oxford University Press, New York, NY.

Van Rossem, R. and Meekers, D. (2000) An evaluation of the effectiveness of targeted social marketing to promote adolescent and young adult reproductive health in Cameroon. *AIDS Education and Prevention*, **12**, 383–404.

Varley, R. C., Tarvid, J., and Chao, D. N. (1998) A reassessment of the cost-effectiveness of water and sanitation interventions in programmes for controlling childhood diarrhoea. *Bulletin of the World Health Organization*, **76**, 617–631.

Wedel, M. and Kamakura, A. (2000) *Market Segmentation: Conceptual and methodological foundations*. Kluwer Academic Publishers, Boston, Dordrecht, London.

Weibe, G. D. (1951–1952) Merchandizing commodities and citizenship on television. *Public Opinion Quarterly*, **15**, 679–691.

World Health Organization (2000) *World Health Report 2000*. World Health Organization, Geneva.

Chapter 8

Evaluating sensitive interventions
Preventing intimate partner violence

Rachel Jewkes

Intimate partner violence affects women in all countries of the world (Watts and Zimmerman 2002). It is an important cause of injury and mortality amongst women as well as a risk factor for a range of physical and mental health problems (Campbell 2002), including HIV infection, depression, pelvic pain and miscarriage. Whilst prevention of intimate partner violence is increasingly seen as an important public health activity, it has only recently moved into the academic mainstream. The range of interventions that have been developed and evaluated is still relatively limited, as governments and donor agencies have yet to allocate levels of resources that are commensurate with the scale of the problem (WHO 2002).

Intimate partner violence has an important impact on health, yet the problem, its implications and interventions extend well beyond the health sector. The WHO World Report on Violence and Health (2002) discusses many of the interventions that have been evaluated. Primary prevention activities include those which promote gender equity and violence reduction in schools; mass media activities to promote a message about the non-acceptability of violence; and risk factor reduction activities such as reducing problem drinking or promoting anger management or non-violent conflict resolution. Secondary prevention activities include the intervention that is often known as screening (and may or may not focus exclusively on the asymptomatic), which involves case identification through sensitive questioning, provision of a simple message about the non-acceptability of violence and referral of cases for further support. Other secondary prevention interventions include legislative measures which criminalize gender-based violence and provide for protection orders and compulsory treatment of offenders; shelters for women; self-help groups; counselling and treatment for men who abuse women and peer education approaches which change community norms on the use of violence and gender relations.

Developing and evaluating such interventions poses certain special challenges. The complex nature of many interventions means that ensuring and demonstrating proper delivery of them may also pose difficulties before outcomes are even assessed. Intimate partner violence takes many highly varied forms, so determining appropriate outcomes, measuring them and attributing effects are considerable challenges.

Challenges of evaluation design

Formative research must precede outcome evaluation so as to be sure that interventions have been thoroughly developed and undergone preliminary testing. Qualitative methods may be particularly useful here. Much can be learnt about an intervention by asking men or women experiencing it how they perceived it and what impact it had on them. This information can also be used later to shape a quantitative evaluation.

The difficulties in delivering effective interventions addressing intimate partner violence are often considerable. In most societies men and women have unequal power and status and these social positions are regarded as reflecting a natural order. It is very difficult to implement an intervention that seeks to build gender equity in relationships if the implementers are unconvinced of the appropriateness of this or if they believe that women are beaten because they deserve it. Interventions should be tested for efficacy in 'ideal' conditions before they are subject to wider roll out and evaluation in other settings. Part of the process of establishing ideal conditions should include giving special attention to the selection of implementers, based on their personal characteristics and ideas about gender relations, and to their training. Qualitative research methods with reports of experiences with the intervention, supported by participant observation or the use of dummy patients, can be useful in these stages.

Expectations of what can be achieved by an intervention should be commensurate with the intervention. In determining realistic outcomes, listening to the women or men who experience the intervention as well as the people who implement the intervention is valuable. An example of an intervention where expectations were not well clarified is that of 'screening'. A review of screening interventions in clinical settings in North America found that most consisted of one session of 1 to 3 hours, which was not enough to achieve sustainable behaviour change in participants who had not previously been introduced to gender and health issues (Garcia Moreno 2002). A more considered approach to addressing the same problem in South Africa, after a careful assessment of the staff backgrounds and skill gaps, resulted in the development of a training course for staff in case identification lasting a total of three days (Jacobs and Jewkes 2002). Evaluations of screening interventions have been criticized for not including long term and health-related outcome measures (Garcia Moreno 2002), but such outcomes may not be realistic considering the intervention's usual design. In the case of screening, given the inevitably long time interval between the first contact with the intervention and leaving relationships or any sustained change in their partner's behaviour, it is not realistic to expect any long term impact. What this intervention could be expected to achieve is:

- To validate a view of the non-acceptability of violence;
- To help change community norms;
- To provide a window of access to support for women;
- To potentially trigger other help-seeking practices.

Evaluation should concentrate on assessing the extent to which these more limited goals are achieved.

Measuring women's experiences of intimate partner violence

Quantitative evaluation of intimate partner violence is challenging, but it has an important role in rigorous assessment of interventions alongside the use of qualitative methods. It is important to consider the range of potential abuse. Apart from physical violence, intimate partner violence also includes sexual and psychological abuse, and all forms of abuse have been found to influence health risks (e.g. WHO 2002; Dunkle *et al.* 2004*a*).

Considerable work has been undertaken internationally to develop best practice in violence research (Ellsberg and Heise 2002) and to create instruments that measure experiences of physical and sexual intimate partner violence in a way which is both locally valid and allows for comparison across settings. For example, the World Health Organization has developed an instrument for its Multi-country study on Women's Health and Gender-based Violence which has now been tested in over a dozen countries (WHO Multi-country Study Core Team 2000). They recommend that questions on physical and sexual abuse focus on discrete acts of violence rather than using broad and potentially charged and subjectively interpreted words. So, for example, a question should be asked about 'kicking' or 'use of a weapon' rather than a general one about 'physical violence or abuse'.

The effects of an act of physical violence linger after the injuries have healed, and often women describe living in a pervasive atmosphere of fear in between the violent acts. There have been some attempts to develop measures of women's subjective experiences of violence and control in relationships that extend beyond the measurement of violent acts. Two notable examples are the Sexual Relationship Power Scale (Pulerwitz *et al.* 2000) and the WEB Scale (Smith *et al.* 1995). Landenburger (1998) described a cycle of episodes of intimate partner violence followed by periods of remorse accompanied by affectionate behaviour, but then followed by tension-building phases before violence is repeated. Most researchers agree that these elements are found in many abusive relationships, although the cycle is rather stylized. This poses a challenge for people who want to evaluate the effectiveness of interventions, as positive perceptions of change in a relationship may merely be a product of data capture during the partner's remorseful (honeymoon) phase. Better practice in evaluation of intimate partner violence would include use of a measure of the frequency of discrete violent acts and a measure of women's subjective experiences.

If frequency of physically or sexually violent acts is used as the outcome measure in an evaluation, the period over which this is measured is critical. If the period of recall is too long, events are forgotten and so there is greater inaccuracy in measurement. Having a period that is too short could lead to exaggeration of the frequency because episodes occurring outside the recall period are erroneously included. Frequency of abuse is problematic as an outcome measure because few women experience physical intimate partner violence on a daily or even weekly basis. For many women, it is much less common. Research in South Africa suggests that approximately a third of women who had ever experienced physical or sexual violence from an intimate partner had only had one episode and that a similar proportion of those experiencing it in the past year have only experienced it once (Dunkle *et al.* 2004*b*). Time since the last act of physical (or psychological or sexual) violence may also be a useful outcome measure, since it is less liable to recall bias and captures a different dimension of experiences from a frequency measure.

Psychological abuse is an important dimension of intimate partner violence but is even more difficult to measure. A key problem is that what constitutes 'psychological abuse' depends on a woman's subjective experiences of her partner's actions (as well as his intentions). There is considerable variation between settings in how these are interpreted. Because of this, enumerating all acts of psychological abuse is probably impossible (unlike the case with physical or sexual abuse where it is more possible to ask about a full range of possibilities). It is not very surprising that there is no substantial body of international opinion on how to define or measure psychological abuse. It is generally agreed that shouting, belittling, verbal abuse and threats of violence are common manifestations, but in some countries other forms of abuse are also common. These may include, for example, taking a partner's earnings, evicting her from home, stalking, bringing home or boasting about other girlfriends, undermining self-esteem, failing to contribute to maintenance or the household, dictating what she wears, or trying to control her behaviour and movements. Moreover, measuring discrete acts of psychological abuse may fail to capture the pervasive atmosphere created by such acts.

While psychological abuse is difficult to measure, it is important that all forms of intimate partner violence that are locally relevant are measured in an evaluation, as interventions which focus on one type – such as stopping the use of physical violence – may result in an increase of other forms, particularly psychological abuse (Holt *et al.* 2002).

Example: Evaluation of the HIV prevention and gender-based violence reduction behavioural intervention Stepping Stones

This intervention is being evaluated in rural South Africa using a randomized controlled trial and qualitative research methods: 2800 men and women aged 17–23 years have been enrolled in the two year study. The following measures of intimate partner violence have been included in the questionnaires for women and (in mirror image) for men:

- 5 items describing psychologically abusive acts by an intimate partner in the past year
- 6 items describing physically abusive acts by an intimate partner in the past year
- 3 items describing sexually abusive acts by an intimate partner in the past year
- Total number of physically and sexually violent episodes in last year
- Date of last physically violent episode and date of last sexually violent episode (to allow computation of time since last episode)
- 13-item relationship control scale adapted from Pulerwitz *et al.* (2000).

In addition, repeated in-depth interviews are being conducted with a subgroup of participants to assess experiences of any change in gender relations more subjectively.

Evaluations of intimate partner violence interventions must take into account the possibility that the intervention may worsen women's relationships. Although some women find that abuse stops when they have the strength to stand up to their partner, others find that such action escalates abuse. This needs to be taken into consideration in intervention design and the design of the evaluation. This will impact on the duration of the study as the short and long-term impact of the intervention may differ. For example a study evaluating the impact on physical intimate partner violence of getting a permanent protection order found no effect at six months but a significant reduction at one year (Holt *et al.* 2002). In this study abuse reported to the police was the outcome measure. In many studies, measures are more subjective and recall is relied upon.

There is the risk that the intervention will differentially influence recall. It could either result in more abusive episodes being recalled because the memory has been jogged, or fewer episodes being recalled if participants were to perceive that to be the socially acceptable answer. This can make it difficult to interpret findings.

Evaluating interventions to reduce men's use of intimate partner violence

For the most part, intimate partner violence involves acts of violence by men directed against women. Women are the focus of many of the secondary prevention interventions, because they need support, but men's behaviour has to change if violence is to be reduced. Interventions that focus on men clearly must be able to measure men's use of violence. Measurement of men's reports of violence has not been studied as much as the reports of women. The validity of men's self-reports is not well established; such reports may well be altered by men's experience of an intimate partner violence prevention intervention. Evaluations of interventions that seek to reduce men's use of violence should include interviews with their female partners, exploring both violent acts and their subjective experiences of violence. Such evaluation becomes more complicated if men have changed partners or are partnerless at the end of the intervention.

Attributing change to interventions

It is difficult to decide what constitutes a positive outcome for intimate partner violence prevention interventions. Clearly, it is important to reduce or end the violence that women experience in their
lives. This is particularly difficult to measure, and difficult to achieve
by a single intervention. The ethical standards that must be followed
in intimate partner violence research may make assessing the outcomes particularly difficult. In evaluating interventions it is impossible to have a true control group. The process of being asked about
intimate partner violence in the interview, with the accompanying
messages about the non-acceptability of violence and the provision of
referral information that must be given to meet ethical standards
(Ellsberg and Heise 2002), are an intervention in themselves. This
intervention, which is provided in the course of the research, may be
as substantial as the intervention being evaluated. This is especially
true in an evaluation of screening by health care workers. In the worst
case this makes rigorous evaluation impossible, in other cases it will
have a substantial influence on estimations of the expected magnitude of effect.

Many of the problems of attributing a cause to an observed behaviour change that have been discussed elsewhere in this book (for
example in the chapter on mass media) pertain to interventions seeking to reduce intimate partner violence. Most women in violent relationships are not able to simply leave them or stop the violence, or
they would probably have already done so. The process of taking
action may be started by that initial contact with an intervention,
a chance to talk with a doctor or nurse, or seeing a billboard message
that women do not need to tolerate such behaviours. The impact of
these, if seen at all, should be expected to evolve along a slow, spi-
ralling and convoluted pathway from there and will include exposure
to other interventions or action promoting experiences. Experience
of non-governmental organizations that help abused women is that
clients often want to test the water when they make their first contact,
talk about problems and get reassurance about themselves, and only
later try forms of interventions such as leaving. Even then, they often
go back to their partner multiple times. Some will try to get other

family members to intervene. They may get a temporary protection order several times, as often they will not go on to having the order made permanent the first time they apply, or they may engage with other legal and social interventions. If women leave a violent relationship, the process often takes several years. Many women do not ever choose to leave, what they seek is for the violence to stop or lessen, and again over time this may happen.

A further problem stems from the fact that most interventions focus on the current relationship, yet it is known that women who date again after experiencing violence often have serially abusive relationships. Ideally evaluations should have long enough follow-up to capture this, but in practice this is rarely made possible due to the limitation of funds and resources needed for such a long follow-up.

Conclusions

Intervention evaluation design must be driven by the research question. 'Are we implementing the intervention as intended?' and must precede the question 'Does the intervention work?' The first question is best answered by qualitative methods and good evaluations will listen carefully to the participants' experiences of the implementation, both for honing the intervention and shaping the evaluation. This process often takes one or more years and should be adequately resourced if interventions are to be well developed before they are tested. In formal quantitative evaluation, those carrying out the evaluation should anticipate that a long-term impact might not be seen until some years after the initial intervention is experienced, in the short term abuse may either escalate or appear to have reduced in frequency.

Evaluations must explore multiple forms of intimate partner violence and consider the subjective experiences of women as well as more objective measures of frequency and severity. Outcomes are more likely to be influenced by exposure to multiple interventions or to important life events. All this suggests the need for long-term experimental community-based research to enable a better understanding of the natural history of gender-based violence and the impact of different interventions to be developed. An ultimate goal for evaluation would be to demonstrate whether concerted efforts to intervene could result in improvements in women's mental and physical health and a reduction in intimate partner violence.

Key points

◆ Interventions must be shown to have been adequately developed and their potential understood before a major evaluation is attempted.

◆ Subjects of an intervention should be interviewed to understand its impact and potential.

◆ Both subjective and objective experiences of intimate partner violence must be measured.

◆ Psychological, sexual and physical intimate partner violence should be assessed as outcome measures.

◆ Interventions with men must include an evaluation of women's views of change in violence.

◆ Attributing change is very difficult and long time frames are needed for thorough evaluations.

References

Campbell, J. C. (2002) Health consequences of intimate partner violence. *Lancet,* **359**, 1331–1336.

Dunkle, K., Jewkes, R., Brown, H., Gray, G., McIntyre, J., and Harlow, S. (2004*a*) Gender-based violence, relationship power and risk of prevalent HIV infection among women attending antenatal clinics in Soweto, South Africa. *Lancet, 363,* 1415–1421.

Dunkle, K., Jewkes, R., Brown, H., Gray, G., McIntyre, J., Yoshihama, M., and Harlow, S. (2004*b*) Prevalence and patterns of gender-based violence and revictimization among women attending antenatal clinics in Soweto, South Africa. *American Journal of Epidemiology.*

Ellsberg, M. and L. Heise (2002) Bearing witness: ethics of domestic violence research. Lancet **359**, 1599–1604.

Garcia Moreno, C. (2002) Dilemmas and opportunities for an appropriate health-service response to violence against women. *Lancet*, **359**, 1509–1514.

Smith, P. H., Earp, J. A., and DeVellis, R. (1995) Measuring battering: Development of the Women's Experience with Battering (WEB) scale. *Women's Health: Research on Gender, Behavior, and Policy*, **1** (4), 273–288.

Holt, V. L., Kernic, M. A., Lumley, T., Wolf, M. E., and Rivara, P. (2002) Civil protection orders and risk of subsequent police-reported violence. *JAMA*, **288**, 585–594.

Jacobs, T. and Jewkes, R. (2002) Vezimfihlo: a model for health sector response to gender violence in South Africa. *International Journal of Obstetrics and Gynaecology*, **78** (Suppl. 1), S51–56.

Jewkes, R., Watts, C., Abrahams, N., Penn-Kekana, L., and Garcia-Moreno, C. (2000) Ethical and methodological issues in conducting research on gender-based violence in Southern Africa. *Reproductive Health Matters*, **8**, 93–103.

Landenburger, K. M. (1998) The dynamics of leaving and recovering from an abusive relationship. *Journal of Obstetric, Gynaecologic and Neonatal Nursing*, **27**, 700–706.

Pulerwitz, J., Gortmaker, S., and DeJong, W. (2000) Measuring sexual relationship power in HIV/STD research. Sex Roles, **42**, 637–660.

Watts, C. and Zimmerman, K. (2002) Violence against women: global scope and magnitude. *Lancet*, **359**, 1232–1237.

WHO Multi-Country Study Core Team (2000) *WHO Multi-Country Study On Women's Health And Life Events Questionnaire version 9. 9.* WHO, Geneva.

World Health Organization (2002) *World Report on Violence and Health*, chapter 4, Violence by intimate partners. World Health Organization, Geneva.

Chapter 9

Evaluating community development initiatives in health promotion

Rachel Jewkes

Community development initiatives involve interaction and engagement with a broadly defined group of people over a period of time to explore their health and social needs and mobilize resources to meet these needs. Very often this involves improving primary health care services or promoting healthier practices. A community development intervention differs from other more individual health promotion approaches, such as peer education, or improvements in treatment or counselling, in important respects. The health impact of the whole project is expected to be greater than the sum of its parts and the process of participation in the initiative is perceived to be beneficial because it is empowering (see also Chapter 6 for a description of community development projects). It is hoped that the processes of participation in a community development project will enable participants to develop skills and competencies which can be applied to areas of life extending well beyond the activities of the project, and will encourage participants to develop social capital – i.e. resources existing because of or arising out of social relationships (Spellerberg 2001) – which in itself is health enhancing (Jewkes and Murcott 1998). When organizations in a community participate in such initiatives, there is an opportunity for impact on the participating organizations. Evaluation of community development initiatives must therefore focus as much on the nature and extent of community involvement in the project (an integral part of process evaluation) as on the outcomes of the component activities and impact in terms of improvements in health.

Evaluations of community development initiatives pose considerable challenges. These stem from the fact that the objectives and activities of an initiative are usually iterative in nature, there may be no predefined end point or criteria for a successful outcome. These challenges compound the methodological problems that are common to other health promotion evaluations, including the need for a mixture of methods, long time frames for health outcomes and difficulties of detecting moderate benefits when communities are small. In addition there is inevitably fluidity in the participant group and fluctuation in the nature of participation. Decisions about who to work with and which projects to work on are strongly influenced by local, and sometimes national, political factors. It is these problems that form the core of this chapter, for whilst the notions of community, participation and power are common currency in health promotion literature, they are amongst the most hotly debated and contested ideas within the social sciences. Their operationalization within community development initiatives poses considerable theoretical and practical difficulties that are important because of the emphasis on process evaluation in this type of health promotion intervention.

Meanings of community

The search for an empirically-based understanding of the nature of community was a major theme in twentieth-century sociology. An overview of the literature can be found in Jewkes and Murcott (1996). By the 1960s, sociologists had come to accept that an agreed and substantiated definition of community could not be attained. Nonetheless the health literature relating to community participation is replete with normatively prescribed definitions. For example, Suliman defines community as 'a group of people with a sense of belonging, with a common perception of collective needs and priorities and able to assume a collective responsibility for collective decisions' (Suliman 1983 p. 407). Adams (1989) states that it should be defined 'geographically or as a community of interest e.g. a street, estate, women's group, black group, pensioner's group'. Frequently those engaged in community participation (e.g. Cutts 1985) have reflected that what might be thought of as a community in definitions like the latter, often do not match up to the former. In practice normative definitions are at best a guide, and those working in the area are forced to continuously adjudicate competing meanings.

Some insights into how this is done can be found in the work of Jewkes and Murcott (1996), who studied community development initiatives in four districts in south east England. They found 28 different types of definition of community within interviews discussing the projects. The constraints of funding and project management required each initiative to have a formal definition, for example 'everyone who lives and works in Westminster' or 'everyone who lives on a housing estate'. This described the boundaries of the community development initiative, and the broad aim of the project was framed in terms of promoting health within this 'community'. Its definition was based on local authority and/or geographic boundaries, which were important for access to resources. This definition was not perceived to be relevant to the daily activities of most of the people working with 'the community'. Instead they constructed 'communities' for these purposes from sub-segments of this community, usually around a defining characteristic which suggested a particular type of need, for example, adolescents in youth clubs might be a community for a drug-use intervention or Kurdish women refugees for activities around women's health services. The relationship between these 'communities' and the formally defined one was described in terms of 'communities within the community'.

Instead of there being one community to consider in an evaluation, there are many. Each activity within a community development initiative will be organized with, and is intended to impact on, a different subset of the population. This must be taken into account in evaluation. For each activity the relevant group must be defined and characteristics of participation and outcomes evaluated with respect to this. Work is often undertaken through organizations that appear to represent a particular group. This is not to say that the formal definition of 'community' is never appropriate to use. Some interventions will be applied to the whole population, and clearly the extent and nature of community participation in the community development initiative overall, must be evaluated with respect to this. What is important is that evaluators question who is the appropriate target group for each aspect of the evaluation, rather than assuming that the formal definition of community is appropriate.

Who participates?

In constructing these smaller 'communities', health promoters implicitly recognize that what may be called a community within a community development initiative is a heterogeneous group with multiple, inter-related axes of difference, including wealth, gender, age, religion, ethnicity and, by implication, power. At times the 'community' may actually be a powerful sector such as district health services or a major local employer. Navarro suggests that a community should be regarded as a set of power relations within which people (and organizations) are grouped (1984). Health promoters working in such environments are continuously faced with choices as to who to work with, be this through accepting an approach from a 'community' or through the deliberate selection of people or organizations as collaborators. These choices inevitably have consequences in terms of the dynamics of power at a local level and ultimately the ability of the initiative to maximize its potential impact in the population.

Steering committee membership and other participant roles

One set of decisions relate to the construction of steering groups for the initiative and often some of the sub-activities of the initiative. Projects may be most easily facilitated if organized through the medium of dominant local stakeholders or 'leaders', who are often most able to mobilize resources and articulate concerns. Yet the poorest and most marginalized are rarely represented amongst them. Working through local power structures may increase the potential impact of a project and its ability to mobilize resources, but it also invites manipulation of it according to the agendas of the powerful. Working outside (and inevitably, at times against) these structures can weaken both the potential impact of the project, as well as invite continued marginalization. Ideally the initiative's steering group should have broad representation, including both the most powerful and marginalized, but in practice this is rarely successfully achieved. Jewkes and Murcott (1998) found that in determining the membership of such steering groups, even amongst representatives of the more marginalized, practical concerns, such as whether someone had a telephone, or was available for daytime meetings, took precedence over all other considerations, including the extent to which different sectors of the population were reflected on the committee or had a mandate to 'represent'. They found the 'community' to be represented almost exclusively by voluntary sector organizations and the representatives drawn from the funded elite of the voluntary sector. Thus even the representatives of the less powerful came from the most privileged quarters of that group. Other studies have shown that participants are usually people of higher income, educational level and occupational group than average (Bates 1983 p. 16).

It is hardly surprising, then, that concern about the representativeness of community representatives is a recurring theme within the evaluation of community development initiatives. Indeed, given the dimensions of difference within the community, it is more surprising that anyone could consider that a small group of people could represent something as diverse as a notion of 'the community' than it is that those who try to do so are regarded as inadequate. Community representatives on steering groups should be chosen and valued for what they have to offer the group rather than perceiving them as representatives of an idealized 'community'. In this way their power bases can be recognized and biases acknowledged, rather than wished away. Representatives can be helped to be more accountable by giving them time to consult their community and ensuring that relevant structures for this are in place.

Whether on the steering committee, or in the project as a whole, its important to recognize that not everyone within communities will be able to participate, nor will everyone be motivated to become involved (Seeley et al. 1992). Even if people are interested they may not be able to give the time. Participation is time-consuming and often those who health promoters want to work with are too busy securing the necessities of life (Agudelo 1983). Considerable efforts are needed to involve marginalized groups. Participating communities are 'made not born'. Unless a commitment to working with the less powerful is part of the process, those who are inaccessible, unorganized and fragmented can easily be left out. Sometimes legitimate decisions must be made to exclude certain groups or individuals. In circumstances of extreme polarization, community development initiatives that have failed to acknowledge the reality of local politics have been turned into arenas for playing out macro-political struggles and have failed (Thornton and Ramphele 1989).

Evaluation and monitoring of who participates, both at a steering committee level and in individual activities within the initiative is essential, as many projects fail to engage non-elite groups (Reidy and Kitching 1986). Unless power dynamics are acknowledged in initiatives, there is a danger that engagement, particularly with more powerful groups, will result in initiatives intended to benefit those with greatest needs being used to their detriment (Nichter 1984).

Nature of participation

Once participation is secured, involvement in the research process is not usually continuous, evenly sustained, or predictable. Participatory theorists have argued that participation can be best described as occurring in different degrees of involvement, ranging from full control by the 'community' through partnership, consultation to information receiving or even manipulation (e.g. Arnstein 1969). In practice, different participants are likely to participate to different degrees and in different ways. One participant may participate differently in different activities of the initiative or different stages of one activity.

Where participation is found to be limited, this is often perceived as primarily attributable to the willingness of those with greater power within the initiative, often the statutory sector, to concede power. It is also true that commitment and interest from community members waxes and wanes over time for a variety of reasons. People may be reluctant to invest their time and energy in the project if it offers little in terms of direct or immediate benefit. Others may enter the participatory process with preconceived ideas of desirable outcomes. When it becomes apparent that these are not project priorities, their enthusiasm may wane. Local people may find that some of the needs that they identify are embraced with more enthusiasm and interest than others. For example, people are often encouraged to identify needs for behaviour change but not for employment. Practitioners need to tread a careful path between generating sufficient interest for participation and not raising false hopes. Identifying honestly the limitations of what can be achieved at the outset is an important part of establishing trust. This takes considerable time.

Evaluation of participation in the project as a whole and in its individual activities must look at the degree of participation, as well as the number and characteristics of the community members who are engaged. It should be done in a sufficiently complex manner to accommodate changes over time in different dimensions of the project. This is important both in ensuring that the objective of participation is achieved and that the extent of participation in activities is taken into account in the evaluation of their outcomes.

Whose agenda dominates?

Many authors (for example Cohen 1985) identify sharing characteristics, experiences or views as a defining feature of community. It is not surprising that people engaged with health promotion do so too. This becomes a problem in community development because a critical distinction needs to be recognized between communities constructed by their members (i.e. those people who we think we share things with) and those constructed by non-members (i.e. people who are assumed to share things). In the course of implementing sets of health promotion activities the boundaries of the 'communities' who are the targets are invariably determined by non-members. The boundaries of sharing are therefore assumed.

Within any local area people associate with one another through multiple networks, they link up in diverse ways around different interests. Isolated axes of difference, such as age or gender, are often insufficient determinants of shared needs for coherent priorities to be identifiable among groups defined in this way. Health promoters find that competing, contested and changing versions of community needs or values emerge according to the way in which their intentions are interpreted by these groups. These not only generate different interpretations, but also reveal different agendas and means for enacting some solutions and blocking others. Caution is needed even when apparently coherent expressions of community needs or priorities are articulated; 'we think . . . ' 'we want . . . ' may reflect a significant distortion of an individual's aspirations. The very act of the 'community' engaging with outsiders necessitates a simplification of their shared experiences into a form and generality that is intelligible to the outsider. This simplification may imply notions of sameness that border on fiction and would not pass within the community (Cohen 1985). In the process of evaluation, health promoters should reflect continuously on whose view is prevailing or whose needs are being expressed, what may be motivating this and what alternative sets of needs and priorities might have been chosen.

A further consequence of assumptions of sharing is a, usually implicit, idea that the benefits of an intervention, particularly the political and other transferable skills derived from participation, will diffuse within the community and in some way impact upon a broader group of people than those who are directly involved. This assumption is almost never evaluated, but the extent to which this occurs should be considered in the evaluation, as it determines the number of people reached through an initiative (halo effect) and this is an important aspect of evaluation (for further discussion of halo effects see Chapter 7).

Does participation impact on the participants?

Much of the literature on community participation assumes that participants will be individuals or representatives of individuals. Yet in many community development initiatives key local stakeholders are involved as organizations or their representatives. In a community development project in South Africa, for example, local employers were included both because they were perceived to have resources which could be accessed for the project and also because they were gatekeepers for a key target group of the community. Representatives of local services, health care and social work may also be included (Campbell 2003). The role of statutory sector organizations and business interests as participants in community development projects has been neglected in theoretical literature. Campbell (2003) has argued that they should be viewed as powerful local forces that can operate to enable or hinder the objectives of community development initiatives. For such organizations to play a constructive role, their participation should accommodate and include the transformation of aspects of their organizations and their work. Engagement in the process of participation should entail some accountability to the steering committee, potential beneficiaries and donors, with a commitment to the propagation of new ideas within all stakeholders participating in the community development initiative as well as the 'target' community. Six principles for successful stakeholding are outlined in the box below, and evaluations should consider the extent to which these are met within a project. This would include the personal characteristics of stakeholder representatives, their position, support for the stakeholder group in terms of management and organizational development, the breadth of stakeholders' constituencies, accountability to these constituencies and the commitment of stakeholders to develop new practices and embrace new ways of working.

Six lessons about stakeholding

1 Stakeholders must understand the philosophy of the multi-stakeholder project management approach, i.e. that existing approaches to the problem are inadequate and that a new approach needs to be forged. This requires transformation of the working practices of the stakeholders' base organizations as well as developing new ways of collaborating.

2 A commitment to innovative approaches is important. Stakeholders must have the power to mobilize their constituencies to support key project activities involving new ways of thinking and behaving.

3 Stakeholder representatives need to be highly motivated individuals with exceptional leadership skills so they can influence their organizations.

4 Stakeholder committees must have access to management skills and organizational development and systems development expertise. These are essential to develop systems to facilitate collaboration of disparate constituencies in innovative approaches.

Six lessons about stakeholding *(Contd.)*

5 Projects need to acknowledge that doctors, nurses and researchers often do not have the expertise to manage complex projects. Stakeholder committees need to draw from a wide range of often excluded groups. including marginalized sectors of the community and front line project staff and develop ways for them to effectively participate and have their views addressed seriously.

6 There needs to be more work to clarify the boundaries of different stakeholder groups. including exactly which interests are represented by each stakeholder. Transparent mechanisms need to be established to ensure that the stakeholders can consult their constituency and be fully accountable to those they represent.

(from Campbell 2003, p. 179)

Conclusions

Community development initiatives are characterized by multifaceted interventions, seeking participation and joint working in the project as a whole as well as in the constituent activities. Evaluation of these projects must also be multifaceted and specifically tailored to each part of the broader initiative. Definition of the population of relevance for each intervention and evaluation of its impact in that group is essential. Evaluation and monitoring of participation are important because the process of participation is perceived to be health generating. Such evaluation should include the impact of participation on major actors in the stakeholder group, and should be undertaken with reference to five questions:

◆ Who participates?
◆ What is the nature of that participation?
◆ Whose agenda dominates?

♦ How does participation impact on participants from all sectors?

♦ How does the participatory process impact on non-participants in the community?

Key points

♦ A consensus on what is community cannot be achieved; it must be defined specifically for each project evaluation.

♦ Targeted efforts must be made to reach disadvantaged groups, otherwise only the more advantaged participate.

♦ Evaluation should acknowledge that consistently high levels of participation by all players are not achievable.

♦ Evaluation should not require that representatives on steering groups are representative, but should consider why they were chosen and whether it was appropriate.

♦ Participatory processes should seek to impact upon all participants and not just those from marginalized groups or individuals from the community.

References

Adams, L. (1989) Healthy cities, healthy participation. *Health Education Journal,* **48**, 178–182.

Agudelo, C. A. (1983) Community participation in health activities: some concepts and appraisal criteria. *Bulletin of the Pan American Health Organization,* **17**, 375–385.

Arnstein, S. (1969) Eight rungs on a ladder of citizen participation. *AIP Journal,* July, 216–224.

Bates, E. (1983) *Health Systems and Public Scrutiny.* Croom Helm, London.

Campbell, C. (2003) *'Letting them Die': Why HIV/AIDS interventions fail.* James Currey, Oxford.

Cohen, A. P. (1985) *The Symbolic Construction of Community.* Routledge, London.

Cutts, F. (1985) Community participation in Afghan refugee camps in Pakistan. *Journal of Tropical Medicine and Hygiene*, **88**, 407–413.

Jewkes, R. K. and Murcott, A. (1996) Meanings of community. *Social Science and Medicine*, **43**, 555–563.

Jewkes, R. and Murcott, A. (1998) Community representatives: representing the 'community'? *Social Science and Medicine*, **46**, 843–858.

Navarro, V. (1984) A critique of the ideological and political positions of the Willy Brandt Report and the WHO Alma Ata Declaration. *Social Science and Medicine*, **18**, 467–474.

Nichter, M. (1984) Project community diagnosis: participatory research as a first step toward community involvement in primary health care. *Social Science and Medicine*, **19**, 237–252.

Reidy, A. and Kitching, G. (1986) Primary health care: our sacred cow, their white elephant? *Public Administration and Development*, **6**, 425–433.

Seeley, J. A., Kengeya-Kayondo, J. F., and Mulder, D. W. (1992) Community-based HIV/AIDS research – whither community participation? Unsolved problems in a research programme in rural Uganda. *Social Science and Medicine*, **34**, 1089–1095.

Spellerberg, A. (2001) *Framework for the Measurement of Social Capital in New Zealand*. Statistics New Zealand, Wellington.

Suliman, A. (1983) Effective refugee health depends on community participation. *Carnets de L'enfance* **2**, 2.

Thornton, R. J. and Ramphele, M. (1989) Community. Concept and practice in South Africa. *Critique of Anthropology*, **9**, 75–87.

Chapter 10

Evaluating the ethics of health promotion
Acquiring informed consent

Dalya Marks

Ethical issues in health promotion are often overlooked. Interventions are often planned, executed and evaluated without any attention being paid to the ethical issues that surround them. There is an assumption that health promotion is good for you and therefore, with many interventions, compliance is expected rather than requested. Furthermore, ethical considerations are rarely included in the overall intervention or programme evaluation. This chapter examines some of the ethical issues surrounding the notions of 'informed consent' and informed decision-making, and highlights some of the broader ethical issues facing health promotion interventions. Interest in these issues has been focused principally in the context of screening pro- grammes, where health promotion initiatives are directed towards identifying high-risk individuals and then putting in place initiatives to change the individuals' behaviour and reduce risk. However, the same important considerations apply to other individually based health promotion interventions, such as immunization, or giving routine malaria prophylaxis to pregnant women.

The model of informed consent requires that participants are provid- ed with unbiased information on the risks and benefits involved in the procedure they have been asked to participate in, and are then free to make the decision on whether or not to participate. Such a model of consent is difficult, and impossible to fully achieve, although guide- lines for providing information prior to consent are available. There are practical problems in delivering the information, but the process of acquiring informed consent also raises concerns among health professionals. Tensions surround the conflicting priorities both to achieve a high programme uptake and to accept that an informed person might decide *not to* participate. In evaluating a health promotion programme, the outcome should not be measured simply in terms of uptake but also in terms of *informed* uptake. Evaluation should include measures of knowledge and empowerment rather than simply acceptance or refusal.

Informed consent and shared decision-making

An individual is entitled to make an informed choice about whether to accept or decline a screening test through provision of the necessary information about the benefits and disadvantages of such a decision (Department of Health 2000, Jepson and Clegg 2000). This process has been described as

> A reasoned choice . . . made by a reasonable individual using relevant information about the advantages and disadvantages of all the possible courses of action, in accord with the individual's beliefs.
>
> (Bekker *et al.* 1999 p. 1)

Whether this adequately describes what patients experience is unclear. Although it corresponds well with common understanding of respect for autonomy within medical ethics, little is known about the effectiveness of involving patients in decisions about their care or the effect that sharing information will have (Entwistle *et al.* 1998). It is assumed that the more a person knows about the disease and the impact of the intervention, the less the psychological distress will be; but this is not supported by evidence and remains to be proven.

Shared decision-making has four elements (Whelan *et al.* 1997). First, it involves at least two participants (a clinician and a participant). Both parties have to build a consensus. Information is shared and an agreement on the course of action is reached together. Shared decision-making is distinct from the paternalistic model in which doctor knows best, but also distinct from the polar opposite, described as a model of informed decision-making. Informed decision-making assumes that the participant will make the decision on his/her own, whereas shared decision-making recognizes the importance of participant preference but includes a role for the health professional who is equipped with the technical knowledge (Coulter 1997). Both the process of the decision-making and the outcome (intervention choice) are shared, which requires shared access to the evidence supporting decisions rather than an abdication of professional responsibility (Coulter 1997). The development of shared decision-making implies that people will want to take on this role.

Guidelines

The General Medical Council in the UK has issued guidelines on what doctors should cover before undertaking a screening procedure (such as a mammogram, test for HIV status, or measurement of blood cholesterol levels) (General Medical Council 1999). The purpose of screening should be explained, as should the likelihood of receiving a positive or negative result, the chance of getting a false positive or false negative result, the risks and uncertainties of the process, and the potential for financial and/or social discrimination. Also, after the test, follow-up plans and the availability of support or counselling services should be discussed. The GMC guidelines do not state how much information should be given, or how it should be conveyed to facilitate informed decision-making.

The UK National Screening Committee also provides guidelines that state:

> There is a responsibility to ensure that those who accept an invitation (to screening) do so on the basis of informed choice, and appreciate that in accepting an invitation or participating in a programme to reduce their risk of a disease there is a risk of an adverse outcome.

> (Department of Health 2000)

Informed choice implies an acceptance that a decision to refuse a test is as valid an outcome as attendance.

Problems with delivery

Little is known about the effects of providing patients with a full account of the risks and benefits involved in the test they have been offered. Not only do we not know how best to provide this information, which can be framed in a number of different ways, we know even less about the effect of providing informed decision-making in terms of uptake (Jepson and Clegg 2000). There is little information available that is based on empirical evidence.

Another important aspect is the ability of the patient group to absorb the information being conveyed. Five and a half million people in the UK have reading difficulties and 22% of the working population have a low level of literacy (Smith *et al.* 1998). This data comes from a study assessing the readability of patient information leaflets in general practice. It cannot be assumed that patients will be able to absorb the messages presented to them in information leaflets. The issue of literacy is even more important in low income countries where the proportions of people who have no formal education, let alone adequate literacy levels, are even higher.

The focus of patient information leaflets tends to be on presentation and readability rather than content, which can lead to inaccurate and misleading information based on unscientific clinical opinion (Coulter 1998). This demonstrates the difficulty in providing appropriate information, and highlights the tension between achieving informed consent and a high uptake of services and questions whether it is feasible, desirable and achievable. Coulter lists the basic ground rules of effective communication. These include the exchange of accurate information, exploration of anxieties or concerns, opportunities for expressing empathy, awareness of treatment options and a negotiation of different views.

It has been suggested that problems might arise when a person is presented with information on the risks and benefits of the intervention as a 'one size fits all' approach (Goyder *et al.* 2000). That is, if all people, regardless of their circumstances (age, sex, religion or cultural background, educational level), are given a uniform package of advice or counselling, this might not take account of individual belief systems. People need to evaluate the information provided on the basis of their own value system or competing priorities, and if the advice package does not take these individual values into account, both patients and health professionals may be faced with conflicting demands. Research is needed to establish what method(s) of conveying information will achieve the desired outcome of realistically presenting a balanced account of the programme's risks and benefits whilst maintaining the objective of maximizing population health gain (or in the case of an intervention, high throughput) (Goyder *et al.* 2000).

New technologies such as interactive CD-ROMs, computer decision tools or the Internet might focus attention further on presentation and readability rather than content, but it is not known whether these media contribute towards the advancement of informed consent or not. It may be that such advances in communication lead to greater highlighting of the uncertainties around medical interventions or outcomes, which in turn may make the patient's decision harder to make. A review of the evidence on presenting risk information has suggested that when patients receive more information, which is more understandable, they may become more cautious in deciding whether to take treatment, comply with interventions or participate in trials (Edwards *et al.* 2001).

The concept of informed decision-making has led to tensions developing between traditionalists and those advocating individual choice. Traditionalists fear that the promotion of individual choice may jeopardize the public's health. They claim that individualism can endanger the goal of the common good and that there is a mutual interdependence between rights and responsibilities. For example, in the UK, following a media-led scare about the safety of the combined measles, mumps and rubella vaccination, many parents chose not to have their children vaccinated. As a result, the proportion of children immunized has fallen to dangerous levels, and there is now a great deal of concern about the possibility of both measles and mumps epidemics. However, Parker argues that the individualism involved in individual decision-making and the promotion of individual choices is *not* incompatible with broader public interest or communitarian values when the shift in power or decision-making from professional to patient incorporates autonomy, alongside rights and responsibilities (Parker 2001).

The tension between respecting individual autonomy, whilst trying to maximize the benefits for the population, has been discussed with reference to a population cardiovascular screening programme (Marteau *et al.* 2002). The traditional public health approach of the programme aimed to achieve population level morbidity and mortality reductions, and in keeping with this, the information provided was brief and highlighted the health *benefits* of participation. Invitations for screening focused on the benefits of such attendance whilst neglecting the potential harms. These 'harms' could be identification of risk factors for coronary heart disease, which would require long term monitoring, adherence to medication and/or lifestyle changes and an awareness of one's susceptibility to a coronary event. In fact, Marteau *et al.* argue that by providing more balanced accounts of what participation might mean, attendance might be reduced, but if those participating are more motivated to adopt the recommendations, the longer-term outcomes could be more favourable; hence population health gain might not be jeopardized, and a programme might be more cost-effective.

Implications of informed consent

The dilemma between individual choice, autonomy and what is considered in the participant's best interests is frequently raised in the literature. If for example, a participant is well informed (presented with the benefits and risks involved), and then makes a decision which the clinician feels is not the right one, the doctor, or health professional providing the information needs to acknowledge that this decision fits within a patient's values, and therefore might be the appropriate choice for the patient (Ashcroft *et al.* 2001). The decision-making process must be contextualized within an individual's environment, recognizing the complex interaction that would be involved when a patient decides to take one course of action rather than another. Sometimes a decision not to undergo further tests would be the appropriate decision for an individual, and thus the decision *not* to present for screening should be accepted as a positive outcome if the objective is to encourage *informed uptake.*

A systematic review explored this concept, examined factors associated with the uptake of screening programmes, and assessed the effectiveness of methods to increase uptake (Jepson and Clegg 2000). Determinants associated with uptake were previous attendance, recommendation by a doctor to attend, age (although it was not clear if being older or younger affected uptake as it differed for different conditions) and education. In terms of what interventions appeared to affect uptake, invitation letters, telephone calls and telephone counselling, and the removal of financial barriers (such as paying for transport and postage) appeared to be effective (effective in terms of increasing uptake of the programme). However, overall, this review found limited evidence on the effects of providing information, and only four of the 190 intervention studies reported giving information on the risks and benefits and only one study evaluated the effect of this knowledge on the decision-making process. The evidence on the effects of different types of information on screening knowledge or uptake is inconclusive. The authors conclude that attempts to increase uptake should be taken in association with efforts to increase *informed* uptake with 'knowledge' as an outcome to measure the decision-making process. They state that all future studies should measure informed uptake as well as *actual* uptake. This requires an acceptance that the outcome of giving information may be that the patient decides against the intervention. This may be against what the clinician feels is the 'sensible' option, but nevertheless will have to be accepted as an outcome in its own right.

Conclusion

A number of factors are important in the consideration of any health promotion intervention aimed at individuals. There is still uncertainty about what is an effective method to convey information, but greater agreement that adequate information should be provided. Similar concerns apply to community-based interventions.

In evaluating health promotion interventions, the ethics of the intervention should be considered, including the acquisition of consent. Outcomes to be evaluated should include informed uptake as well as actual uptake of an intervention. If an individual decides that on the basis of the information provided, they do not wish to participate in the intervention, that should be regarded as a considered and appropriate decision based on the information provided. It must be accepted that individuals make decisions based on their own beliefs and values, as well as their own perception of the risks involved with accepting or declining an intervention. Outcomes should not only measure throughput, or response rates, but also factors such as knowledge or empowerment. These might help to understand the acceptability and appropriateness of a programme.

Finally time and resource constraints are a real barrier, if the objective of informed choice is to be realized. However, providing an intervention within an informed choice paradigm has the potential of being more cost-effective than if conducted within a traditional public health paradigm if it results in people more willing to present for screening and more motivated to alter their health behaviours.

Key points

- Participants have the right to a full explanation of the risks and benefits of an intervention before consenting to participate.
- Providing adequate information requires investment of time and resources.
- If, after assessing this information provided, an individual decides not to participate, that decision must be respected.
- In evaluating health promotion interventions, informed uptake rather than throughput should be measured.

References

Ashcroft, R., Hope, T. *et al.* (2001) Ethical issues and evidence-based patient choice. In A. Edwards and G. Elwyn *Evidence-based Patient Choice: Inevitable or impossible?* Oxford, Oxford University Press.

Bekker, H., Thornton, J. G. *et al.* (1999) Informed decision making: an annotated bibliography and systematic review. *Health Technology Assessment*, 3 (1), 1–156.

Coulter, A. (1997) Partnerships with patients: the pros and cons of shared clinical decision-making. *J. Health Serv. Res. Policy*, 2 (2), 112–121.

Coulter, A. (1998) Evidence-based patient information: Is important, so there needs to be a national strategy to ensure it. *BMJ*, 317, 225–226.

Department of Health (2000) *Second Report of the National Screening Committee.* DH, London.

Edwards, A., Elwyn, G. *et al.* (2001) Presenting risk information – a review of the effects of 'framing' and other manipulations on patient outcomes. *Journal of Health Communication,* **6,** 61–82.

Entwistle, V. A., Sheldon, T. A. *et al.* (1998) Evidence-informed patient choice. Practical issues of involving patients in decisions about health care technologies. *Int J Technol Assess Health Care,* **14** (2), 212–225.

General Medical Council (1999) *Seeking Patients' Consent: The ethical considerations.* GMC, London.

Goyder, E., Barratt, A. *et al.* (2000) Telling people about screening programmes and screening test results: how can we do it better? *Journal of Medical Screening,* **7,** 123–126.

Jepson, R., Clegg, A. *et al.* (2000) The determinants of screening uptake and interventions for increasing uptake: a systematic review. *Health Technology Assessment,* **14** (14), 1–123.

Marteau, T. M. and Kinmouth, A. L. (2002) Screening for cardiovascular risk: public health imperative or matter for individual informed choice? *BMJ,* **325,** 78–81.

Parker, M. (2001) The ethics of evidence-based patient choice. *Health Expectations,* **4** (2), 87–91.

Smith, H., Gooding, S. *et al.* (1998) Evaluation of readability and accuracy of information leaflets in general practice for patients with asthma. *BMJ,* **317,** 264–265.

Whelan, T., Gafni, A. *et al.* (1997) Shared decision-making in the medical encounter: what does it mean? (or it takes at least two to tango). *Soc Sci Med,* **44** (5), 681–692.

Chapter 11

Evaluating mass media approaches

Kaye Wellings and Wendy Macdowall

Broad spectrum interventions, intended to reach the general population, make use of mass communicational approaches such as TV, radio, press, billboard posters and leaflets. These media are important sources of health information. Not everyone can be reached through community approaches, and high profile communication can reach hidden groups within the general population. Box 1 highlights some of the roles that the mass media can fulfil.

Evaluation is particularly important in the case of mass media interventions because of the high costs involved. Yet the problems inherent in evaluation of all health promotional activities are exacerbated in broad spectrum approaches. The major strength of the mass media (their ability to reach a wide audience) paradoxically presents the greatest challenge for evaluation. Whereas the target

Box 1 The role of mass media

Mass communicational approaches can:
- Reach a wide audience
- Reach hidden groups within the population
- Place the health issue on the public agenda
- Legitimate interventions at other levels
- Trigger other initiatives.

audience of an intervention using a formal educational or clinical setting is more easily followed up, surveillance of the mass audience is more difficult. There is less control over the destination and reception of preventive messages and thus they may fail to reach audiences for which they were intended, or they may reach audiences for which they were not intended and be misconstrued. Furthermore, mass media interventions may have unintended consequences over which health promotion agencies have little control.

Two important themes are of particular concern in the context of mass media interventions:

Observed effects will be smaller

Broad spectrum interventions do not target high risk individuals, who have greater scope for change. Change at the level of a large and undifferentiated population is likely to be smaller.

Effects are more difficult to attribute to mass media intervention

Attributing outcomes to a specific intervention is complicated where mass communicational techniques are used. An effective campaign will have an effect far beyond its original remit, creating media discussion, providing the impetus for local efforts, and so on. The effects of the intervention are not easily distinguished from other events concurrent with it or subsequent events triggered by it.

The scope of interventions: individual change and social diffusion

The strength of mass media, according to some, lies in helping to place issues on the public agenda and in legitimating local efforts, raising consciousness about health issues, and conveying simple information (RUHBC 1989, Tones *et al.* 1990). What the mass media do less effectively is to convey complex information, teach skills, shift attitudes and beliefs and change behaviour in the absence of other enabling factors.

Two models are applicable in the evaluation of mass media interventions. The first, the 'risk factor' or epidemiological model, is principally concerned with changing individual health-related behaviour, based on the premise that this will change health status. The second, the 'social diffusion' model, has more to do with the process of intervention and its catalytic effect, and the interaction between the component parts (Rogers 1983). If mass media interventions are effective, it is likely to be because they activate a complex process of change in social norms rather than because they directly change the behaviour of individuals.

An explicit objective of many mass media campaigns, then, is to change the social context and to effect a favourable climate in which interventions could be received. The college principal/publican/garage proprietor, previously doubtful about the propriety of installing a condom machine in his sixth form college/pub/garage feels reassured and validated by a government-backed mass media campaign promoting condom use. The young person, motivated to use condoms by the same campaign, is further encouraged to do so by their ready accessibility in the college/pub/garage in which he studies/drinks/buys petrol. This is sometimes known as 'diffusion acceleration'.

The discrete contribution of different components is difficult to assess. Influences on our behaviour are multiple and are as likely to counteract, as to be in unison with, health advice. The biggest changes in behaviour, and hence in health status, are likely to come about through forces other than public education. For example, smoking behaviour is determined by the price of cigarettes, by restrictions on smoking in public places and by voluntary impositions of bans (e.g. by a member of household).

Because of the high cost of use of the mass media, a campaign of short duration can consume a large proportion of the funds available for preventive interventions. A valid aim, therefore, may be to prompt coverage of the campaign by the free media.

The evaluation process: stages of research

Evaluation research begins with a *developmental component*, in which the potential for intervention in any health problem is described, along with (wherever possible) identification of factors that might facilitate or obstruct the delivery. This is followed by a *formative evaluation* in which the candidate intervention is pre-tested. During the course of the delivery of the programme a *process evaluation* is undertaken (see also Chapter 6) and finally, an *outcome evaluation* is carried out, which examines effects, effectiveness and efficacy (see Chapter 5 for a discussion of effectiveness and efficacy). If effectiveness is demonstrated and the service continues, routine monitoring and audit subsequently ensure quality of service delivery and continued efficacy.

A circular process

Development of the research and evaluation process is optimally seen not as linear, but circular, i.e. data from the outcome stage of evaluation will feed back into further development of the intervention, closing the loop. Subsequent generations of programmes will benefit from insights into the effectiveness of the last. An important function of evaluation is to provide a means of detecting and solving problems and planning for the future. Providing retrospective feedback on success or failure at the end of an intervention provides guidance when it is too late to do anything about it. Ideally, the process should be continuous, tracking the progress of initiatives over time and feeding back information that can help operational decision-making, although in some situations this may not be possible or desirable (for further discussion of this issue see Chapter 6).

Formative research

Formative research involves exploratory work to guide the design of the intervention. An important component of formative research is the pretesting of materials, as there is potential for messages to be misunderstood. It is important to know whether an intervention failed in its mission because it was not heard, or because it was not understood. Formative research, which typically uses focus groups, is useful in checking that an audience understands the language and images used.

Example: formative research

A series of AIDS public service announcements run by the UK Health Education Authority in spring 1988 aimed to convey the message that adoption of risk reduction practices needs to be universally applied because of the difficulty of distinguishing between those with and without the virus. The advertisement reproduced here (Fig. 11.1) attempted to show that there were rarely visible symptoms of AIDS and that those with HIV have the same facial features as those without. No problems in relation to clarity of the message were revealed during pretesting, but independent research by academic media analysts revealed considerable misinterpretation, with some people believing the advertisement was attempting to convey an accurate impression of what someone with HIV looked like (Kitzinger 1991).

Example: unexpected negative effect

A particularly controversial press advertisement, with the message that we should take not the numbers of people with AIDS as an indication of the scale of the problem, but those with HIV, posed the question 'What is the difference between HIV and AIDS?' and provided the answer 'Time'. Pre-testing showed the advertisement to convey the intended message effectively. The pre-testing research was conducted among the target audience of those who were uninfected, and could not predict the ensuing storm of protest from people with HIV. It proved an insensitive message with dire consequences for those affected, and was consequently withdrawn. Formative evaluation needs to take place with both target and non-target groups.

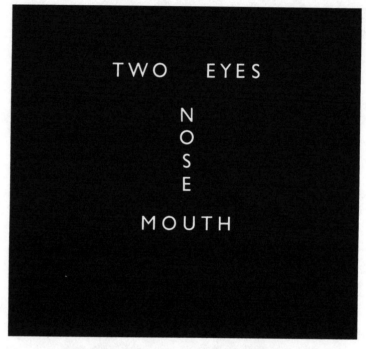

**HOW TO RECOGNISE SOMEONE WITH HIV
(THE VIRUS THAT LEADS TO AIDS).**

We all know how devastating the effects of AIDS can be.

But what are the signs of the Human Immunodeficiency Virus, the virus that leads to AIDS?

The fact is, a person can have HIV for years without the signs developing. During this time they may look and feel perfectly healthy.

But through sexual intercourse, they can pass on the virus to more and more people.

Already there are many thousands of people in this country who are unaware that they have the virus.

Obviously the more people you sleep with the more chance you have of becoming infected. But having fewer partners is only part of the answer.

Safer sex also means using a condom, or alternatively, having sex that avoids penetration.

HIV is now a fact of life.

And while infection may be impossible to recognise, fortunately it is possible to avoid.

AIDS. YOU'RE AS SAFE AS YOU WANT TO BE.

Fig. 11.1

The formative phase of evaluation aims to anticipate possible unforeseen outcomes. These are often favourable. For example, as a result of AIDS education using mass media interventions, the ruling on TV advertising of condoms was changed in several countries, including France, the UK and Ireland (Wellings and Field 1996). But they may also be unfavourable (substitution effect, see Chapter 7).

Process evaluation

Research should be capable of revealing not only *whether* a campaign has succeeded or not but *why*, so that the findings can be used to guide future developments. Process evaluation is often narrowly conceived in terms of measuring 'dose' or exposure – either objectively in terms of the extent to which the campaign was aired (number of TV spots; broadcasting times; frequency and duration; audience figures; numbers of posters/leaflets displayed) or subjectively (TV spots seen; time spent watching; time spent reflecting; level of interest) and in this sense more closely resembles audit.

While outcome evaluation focuses on the goals of a programme, process evaluation is important in providing insights into what factors may hinder or facilitate their achievement (see Chapter 6). Potentially favourable effects of a campaign can be seriously attenuated by an adverse response from the public. By definition and design, exposure to the mass media is universal. Tailoring messages to specific target groups is less easily achieved and problems of social and political acceptance can arise where messages are seen by those for whom they were not intended. Process evaluation also has valuable potential in helping to uncover unintended consequences of intervention.

Process evaluation must take account of the journalistic backdrop against which the campaign is launched. Journalistic coverage of a campaign in the free media will influence the way in which the campaign is received by the public, and may mediate between the originators of a campaign and the intended audience, influencing the selective receipt of messages.

Example: the influence of journalistic coverage

An illustrative example is to be found in the mass media campaign executed as part of the government's Teenage Pregnancy Strategy in 2000, aimed at reducing the under-18 conception rate and reducing social exclusion among young parents (Wellings *et al.* 2001). The designers of the campaign were careful to include in the series of magazine advertisements a hierarchy of messages, aimed at increasing resistance to peer pressure to have sex, encouraging contraception, and changing the social norms governing early motherhood. The campaign, however, was leaked in the press in advance of its launch in young people's magazines. Instead of displaying the complete portfolio of advertisements, journalists focused exclusively on those empowering young women to have sex when they were ready (see the headlines illustrated). This campaign came to be known thereafter as the 'Virgin campaign' and the tracking survey monitoring the views of young people showed recall of this component to be higher than for any other component in the campaign.

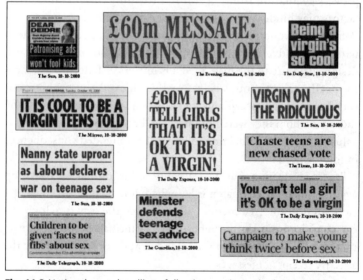

Fig. 11.2 National press headlines following unplanned advance publicity given to the teenage pregnancy campaign: October 2000.

Box 2 Specific issues to be addressed in process evaluation include:

- How well were resources allocated and disseminated?
- Were there any adverse side effects of the intervention?
- Was there harmony between the aims of health promotion and the needs of clients?
- Were there social and political dynamics that interfered with the ways in which health educational messages were received and responded to?
- Were there alliances between different interventions or environmental factors that enhanced outcomes?

Outcome evaluation

Two key criteria for outcome evaluation are the size of effect and the possibility of attributing the outcome to the intervention. On both of these criteria, mass media work is problematic for evaluation.

1 Size of effect

The size of the expected effect is often not specified in the intervention plan, but a vital question is how large the effect has to be in order to make the case for the intervention having worked. Gains made in the case of mass media interventions may be modest for a variety of reasons.

The size of the target population

Effects will be smaller where the target group is a large and heterogeneous mass.

The nature of outcome measures or end points

Changes may be small because the wrong level of objectives has been chosen. Where measures of morbidity and mortality are used as outcomes in interventions aimed at the general population the sample needs to be impossibly large, and the scale of effect may still be too small to interpret.

The scope of the intervention

Little effect may be seen because the end points are too narrowly conceived in terms of individual behaviour. Procedures need to be developed which attempt to measure effectiveness in terms of changes wrought in the social context.

The time scale

The time scale looked at may be too short. Health promotional efforts must be of long duration to have significant effects; despite being small scale, initial differences may be sustainable. The 30-year anti-smoking campaign in the United States is an excellent example of the potential of such sustained efforts.

Some of these issues are dealt with below, under the heading 'Selection of indicators/outcome measures'. Although difficult to interpret, small effects may be of greater consequence where large numbers of people are involved and, even if unpromising when looked at from an individual perspective, can be important in public health terms (see Chapter 3). It is at the level of subgroup activity that achievements become observable, hence the importance of disaggregating data by groups of interest (segmentation – see Chapter 7).

2 Attributing outcome to intervention

A major challenge in assessing the effectiveness of mass media approaches to prevention is that of attributing outcome to intervention, that is, ensuring that the apparent observed effects are truly the outcome of public education campaigns and not the result of a priori differences or differential exposure to something else, such as the mass media generally or local preventive interventions.

Hybrid interventions seem to work better than those with only one component, and the success seems to lie in the interaction effects between component parts. A valid goal for an intervention may be to accelerate trends in already existing behaviour rather than initiate new trends. The effects may be enhanced by synergy; where there are multiple coinciding influences on behaviour, the outcome is likely to be more marked.

'Background noise' is often considered problematic in the context of outcome evaluation. The task of outcome evaluation is to look at the extent to which a mass media intervention is successful in harnessing environmental influences to its aims. Instead of trying to disentangle the variables, efforts need to be made to quantify the interaction effects. It may be beyond the power of an evaluation to determine which elements of the programme were effective. Moreover, it is likely to be misleading to attribute, to a particular focused action, an effect that may well have been the product of a complex mobilization producing norm change. Evaluation efforts need to find ways of measuring the catalytic effect of mass media interventions.

Selection of indicators/outcome measures

Outcome evaluation requires the use of indicators by which the outcomes can be measured. Outcome indicators should be determined by the objectives of interventions, and lack of clarity regarding the objectives of mass media interventions is a common problem in evaluation. If objectives are set at an inappropriate level this can threaten the apparent success of the intervention.

Outcomes relating to proximate points along the causal pathway – awareness of risk, intention to change, modification of attitudes – are more feasible to measure but less attractive in terms of 'proof' of effectiveness, while distal endpoints are more attractive in terms of scientific rigour, but success in achieving these goals will be remote. In most cases, the proximate outcome variable in the biomedical model will be the adoption and maintenance of behaviours that reduce risk and these may constitute the indicators themselves (e.g. condom use, increased uptake of immunization, change in drinking/ smoking habits). Intermediate outcomes might include measures such as serum cholesterol levels and weight, and relate more indirectly to the goals of intervention. The more distal outcomes – incidence of disease or mortality – are not sensitive indicators for the general population, for reasons already discussed.

In practice, a variety of outcome variables is needed, some proximate to the intervention, some intermediate, others more distal. The social diffusion model of health promotion has implications both for the size of the effect needed, and for attributing outcome to intervention. It may be that the effects achieved appear small, but they may prove sustainable because the intervention has triggered a process of diffusion. Therefore a time element needs to be built into the evaluation.

Measuring unintended consequences

Operating within the narrow bounds of a goal-directed model of evaluation will miss identifying possible adverse outcomes. Prior identification and definition of all the outcome variables may result in unforeseen and unintended effects going unrecognized and unrecorded.

Selection of research design

The question 'What are the methodological approaches which will allow us to support or reject claims of success?' follows logically from the question of how success can be measured. Some would argue that the only legitimate goal of evaluation is to assess effectiveness using experimental methods. Randomized controlled trials (RCTs) are rigorous methods of evaluation, but they are not applicable in every case. The success of the experimental approach depends on being able to ensure that observed differences in outcomes do not arise from factors other than the intervention under investigation. Added to the problems of RCTs identified in Chapter 5, there are others that are either unique in the case of mass media interventions, or accentuated by mass media interventions.

The broader the intervention, the more global its remit, the more far reaching its effects, the greater the interaction with other social forces and movements (and ironically the more interesting the outcome), the less amenable it is to evaluation by a RCT. Some of the biggest influences on health-related behaviours and health status occur at national levels. Experimental evaluations are poorly suited to interventions aimed at changing the social context. There are several problems of research design for mass media interventions.

Generalizability

Campaign effects may be dependent on local circumstances that may not be generalizable to other areas or in the future.

Specificity

Experimental and quasi-experimental designs are difficult to apply to mass media campaigns because by definition virtually everyone is exposed to them.

Comparison group

Mass media interventions have problems identifying and maintaining the integrity of a comparison or control group. Many people and behaviours are not amenable to random allocation.

Size of effect

The tendency to use relatively high discount rates (see Chapter 4) in the evaluation of health programmes does not favour health promotion programmes using the mass media. Only small effects are likely to be seen. Where there is a great deal of background communication going on, the intervention may provide only a very small increment.

Contamination

The image of pristine treatment and control communities associated with the notion of the controlled trial is a false one. Trials attempting to give a communication treatment to one place and not to a neighbouring place ignore the social process at work.

Practical, ethical and, in some cases, economic obstacles may also impede the implementation of experimental strategies. The options in terms of experimental approaches that can be applied to the evaluation of mass media interventions include:

♦ Lagged exposure or phased implementation (staggering interventions over time);

♦ Area comparisons (comparing areas with and without interventions); and

♦ The application of media weight bias (comparing populations exposed to media interventions with those not so exposed).

Alternative approaches

There is little point in finding out whether an intervention works better than another or none at all, until we have first established what effects it has and whether there are, in addition to those intended, effects that are unintended and possibly adverse. If the intervention fails to achieve the goals set for it, the question of whether it did so more cost-effectively than another intervention or none at all will be irrelevant (see Chapter 4 for a discussion of measuring cost-effectiveness). Programmes using the mass media should be evaluated with a methodology that respects their character and the way they work, but is credible enough to influence policy decisions. An eclectic approach to research and evaluation is called for; in the words of the late Geoffrey Rose, we need researchers with 'clean minds and dirty hands'. Alternative approaches, including natural experiments, correlated time series and other non-experimental and quasi-experimental approaches are needed.

Measures of effect

Several methods have been used to measure effects and effectiveness.

Retrospective reporting

In this, respondents are simply asked if they have gained in knowledge, changed their attitudes or modified their behaviour. This method may be the only one available in many cases, yet, because of the absence of baseline data, suffers from biases introduced by desirability response and recall difficulties.

Longitudinal designs

These have advantages over a cross-sectional design and are more appropriate to understanding the process of behaviour change. Panel studies, where the same group of people are questioned repeatedly over time, have disadvantages of attrition yet these disadvantages may be balanced by the advantages of being able to track changes in behaviour in the same individuals over time.

Time series data

Evaluation of effectiveness typically uses a pre- and post-test design and these methods are less complex and less costly than RCTs. Time series data use narrative to make the case for observed effects being attributable to the intervention, that is, the equivalent of 'telling a story with data'. Ideally before and after intervention data are needed. Such studies offer some improvement over one shot studies but are still susceptible to desirability response and provide no assurance that what is being measured is the effect of a particular intervention and not a generalized response to the health issue.

Correlated time series

Correlated time series data using pre- and post-test data and statistical modelling techniques, help trace the causal pathway to the objectives, identifying intervening valuables and also control for a number of problems of inference. Strength of effect after controlling for confounding is taken as credible evidence that the intervention was causing the effect. Structural equations, used to examine the direct effect of the intervention, and the indirect effect on intervening variables though the use of regression models, are able to assess the strength of each of the factors.

Knowledge attitude and behaviour surveys

Survey investigation is the mainstay of data collection procedures. Typically, knowledge attitude and behaviour (KAB) surveys are used to investigate exposure to, recall and comprehension of campaign messages and self reported behaviour change. KAB surveys have limitations in the extent to which they can monitor changes wrought in the social context, since their focus is on the individual. They also present problems of validity and reliability and are susceptible to social desirability response.

Triangulation

One solution to the problem of bias in the collecting process has been to attempt to triangulate results, or to cross-validate against other data sources that might provide more objective measures of behavioural change. A good deal of information is available in this respect at relatively low cost and might include a selection from the following: sales figures (of, for example, cigarettes, alcohol, condoms, low-fat spreads), subscriptions to exercise classes, health clubs; immunization uptake; screening uptake e.g. mammography, HIV test data, helpline statistics, morbidity and mortality data and media reports. The combination of behavioural and clinical measures also offers potential for triangulation, helping to verify inferences drawn from self-reported data, despite methodological and scientific difficulties.

Media analysis

As noted above, programmes may work because they activate a complex process of change in social norms rather than because they produce behaviour change directly at the level of the individual. Media analysis provides a valuable indicator of changes in the social context. This requires the use of a reputable media cuttings audit agency, or assiduously keeping a cuttings file. Where the intervention is under trial in one region, such that one area receiving the intervention is compared with another, which does not, local media audit is particularly important.

Independence of the evaluation team

The choice of agency to carry out the evaluations is pivotal in determining the quality of the data produced, the manner in which it was used and its impact on future campaigns. There is clearly a political dimension of evaluation, since it may show projects as not as effective as the originators believed they would be. Inevitably, where those commissioning the evaluation are also responsible for the campaigns, it is more difficult to ensure objectivity and impartiality.

Key points

Evaluation of mass media health promotion interventions should take account of the fact that such approaches:

- Have effects beyond their original remit.
- Influence the social context.
- Reach groups and individuals outside of the target groups.
- May have unintended effects.
- Need to utilize a range of evaluative methods.

References

Kitzinger, J. (1991) Judging by appearances: Audience understandings of the look of someone with HIV. *J. Comm. and App. Psych*, **1** (2), 155–163.

Rogers, E. (1983) *Diffusion of Innovations*. The Free Press, New York.

RUHBC (Research Unit in Health and Behavioural Change) (1989) *Changing the Public Health*. Chichester, John Wiley and Sons.

Tones, K., Tilford, S., and Robinson, Y. (1990) *Health Education, Effectiveness and Efficiency*. Chapman and Hall, London.

Wellings, K. and Field, B. (1996) *Stopping AIDS. AIDS/HIV and the mass media in Europe*. Longman and the European Commission, New York.

Wellings, K., Grundy, C., and Kingori, P. (2001) *Press Coverage of the Young People's Campaign, October 2001: Report prepared for the Department of Health*. London School of Hygiene and Tropical Medicine, London.

Chapter 12

Evaluating the dissemination of health promotion research

Gillian Lewando-Hundt
and Salah Al Zaroo

The dissemination of health promotion research to policy makers, practitioners and users is essential if the gaps between research policy and practice are to be bridged. The findings of research are not the property of research scientists, the funders, or the respondents in the research. Rather, they are part of a shared body of knowledge that cumulatively leads to a better understanding of health promotion.

All too often outside researchers collect information from indigenous experts, publish academic papers that benefit their career and fail to disseminate and share findings with the community that created these findings through their participation. This is an issue of research ethics concerning indigenous and users' rights to the knowledge and benefits of research which should be considered in all settings and regions.

Despite its importance, research dissemination is often poorly resourced and not evaluated. There are papers arguing for dissemination and even arguing the importance of evaluating it (Potvin 1996, Green and Johnson 1996), but there are few published examples of evaluations. Without evidence of whether strategies of disseminating research are effective, it is likely that ineffective strategies will be pursued or effective strategies will be overlooked.

This chapter will begin by examining definitions of dissemination and will then look at how research is disseminated into policy and practice and to users. The focus then moves on to an exploration of the barriers to dissemination and identifies ways of overcoming them, before finally discussing ways of evaluating dissemination.

Definitions of dissemination

Sometimes a differentiation is made between the process of diffusion and dissemination, with diffusion defined as the spread of new knowledge to a defined population, via channels, over time, and dissemination defined as deliberate efforts to spread an innovation. Rogers (1983) however, views diffusion and dissemination as interchangeable terms. In this chapter we will define dissemination as 'dissemination is about the communication of innovation, this being either a planned and systematic process or a passive and unplanned diffusion process'(Crosswaite and Curtice 1991 p. 3).

Communication of knowledge through the dissemination of research findings is a key mechanism for the growth and development of a discipline. Health promotion is no exception to this. If anything, the process of dissemination is more crucial to health promotion than other disciplines because of the guiding principles of participation, empowerment, and equity that underpin it.

Five types of transactions occur when disseminating research and information in relation to health promotion programmes (King *et al.* 1998). Such dissemination encourages:

1 Information sharing about a new programme or finding;

2 Support for the relevance of a new programme or policy;

3 Decision-making to adopt a new idea;

4 Changing practices to implement a new idea or programme;

5 Maintenance of a new practice or policy.

In evaluating dissemination we can distinguish between process evaluation, where the process of how and why transactions occur, or do not occur, is traced, and outcome evaluation, which measures to what extent these changes are achieved. A further delineation can be made in terms of which arena the dissemination is being aimed at – policy, practice, or users.

Disseminating research into policy

There are four models that are generally referred to when discussing the dissemination of research to policy makers (Crosswaite and Curtice 1994):

1 The rational model;
2 The limestone model;
3 The gadfly model;
4 The insider model.

The *rational model* assumes that it is enough to make information available for it to be incorporated into policy making. This rarely, if ever, happens. It is argued by others (Richardson *et al.* 1990) that research informs policy making indirectly and the *limestone model* is more often cited. This model postulates that research findings trickle down into policy making rather as water trickles down through porous limestone, circuitously and slowly. The *gadfly model* places as much emphasis on the dissemination of results as on the research itself, so there are meetings to feedback results to an advisory group, to the media, and to funders, and the publication of findings in a variety of reports and publications which address a range of audiences. Finally, the *insider model* operates when the researchers have links with those inside government or international and national agencies and are therefore able to adapt the presentation of research findings to address policy concerns.

Disseminating research into practice

The practice of health professionals should be informed by the findings of research. Continuing education to health professionals can be delivered in several forms.

Face-to-face interventions

Face-to-face interventions can include seminars, workshops, and one to one meetings including formal supervisions.

Guidelines

Clinical guidelines are defined as systematically developed statements that assist in decisions on appropriate health care for specific conditions. Guidelines can equally well be developed to guide health promotion practice and there is evidence that explicit guidelines improve clinical practice in almost all cases (Grimshaw and Russell 1993).

Newsletters

Newsletters can be on provided on tape, CD, or paper. For example The Safe Motherhood newsletter, funded by the World Health Organization, is distributed free in a variety of languages to practitioners in maternal health internationally.

Evaluation of the use of the Internet as a medium for the delivery of information to health professionals is in its infancy, but this will undoubtedly become an increasingly important source of information for professionals and practitioners, and will require evaluation.

Dissemination of research to participants or service users

Research participants and users of services have a right to be informed about research findings, particularly when they have provided information for the research studies. However, funding for disseminating the findings to participants or service users is rarely provided as part of a research project.

The informed user can be a constructive influence on policy and practice. Today, many funding bodies require researchers to set out their strategies for dissemination and user engagement. One mechanism to ensure some dissemination of research to users is the establishment of a consultative group for the coordination of the dissemination of findings. Consultation takes many forms and can be open and public, for example, in community meetings, or can be through nominated or elected committees. Dissemination to existing NGOs or community groups is also a way of reaching a wider lay audience. This is time-consuming and sometimes delicate, but is worthwhile if research findings are to affect people's lives. Written booklets of information in local languages are often prepared. If meetings with community groups to discuss the material accompany such booklets, then the dissemination will be more effective and the recommendations can be discussed and action plans formulated.

Collaboration between researchers and participants: action research

If a participative research approach is developed, with input from users at different stages of the research process, it is likely that users will develop ownership of the research recommendations and results. The example in Box 1 illustrates this.

Example: Participatory research in water and sanitation improvement

The *Hygiene Evaluation Procedures (HEP) Handbook* was developed in response to practitioner's demand for guidelines on how to incorporate social and cultural considerations in the design of improved water supply, sanitation and health promotion interventions. The handbook tackles the issue of participation of the researched by outlining three basic types of participation. Extractive participation (where researchers merely extract information and disappear) is discouraged in favour of consultative and interactive participation. Moreover, the methods/tools described in the handbook require the investigator to double check and cross-check data by presenting it back to the study population for verification. In this way, their feedback on findings becomes part of the investigation process. This is a basic feedback mechanism to put in place if the final results are to be used by those most concerned, that is, the study population whose practices

Example: Participatory research in water and sanitation improvement *(Contd.)*

health workers and others are trying to influence and change for the better.

The draft *HEP Handbook* was field-tested in different sites through consultative participation of intended users. Once in print, the dissemination process of the handbook and the approach it propagates has continued with seminars, talks and training workshops for training of trainers. There is an evaluation sheet at the end of the book for users to fill in (Almedom *et al.* 1997).

One strategy which takes cognisance of the important role of professional knowledge is practitioner based research or action research with professionals and research scientists. Action research is problem-centred research bridging the gap between theory and practice. Unlike academic research, action research builds utilization strategies into overall research design. Involving professionals in practitioner based action research is also an effective mechanism for ensuring the dissemination and acceptance of research findings. Others have called action research with professionals 'practitioner-based research'. There have been a number of studies undertaken by practitioners to establish the needs of users of their services and the Example box below gives two examples.

Example: Practitioner-based action research in the field of learning difficulties

A study in Coventry, England on the needs of people with learning difficulties involved a team of practitioners including a community psychiatric nurse, two social workers, two nursery nurses, and one translator of Asian languages. The professionals learnt how to carry out research and then presented their findings to management,

Example: Practitioner-based action research in the field of learning difficulties *(Contd.)*

to the families involved in the research and to their colleagues. The project resulted in the establishment of a self-help group for families and in some changes in policy and practice, such as regular benefit checks for families with children with learning difficulties.

A similar study of the family needs of children with learning difficulties, with the team of a Child Development Centre in southern Israel, resulted in the team advocating changes to the service they offered. They recommended and partially implemented integrated appointments, benefit checks, more focus on parental concerns and more provision being given by Arabic-speaking staff (Lewando-Hundt *et al.* 1995).

There are many further examples of action research which involve the active participation of practitioners (Hart and Bond 1995), and this model has much to offer.

In addition, participatory action research with community members promotes a dialogue and interchange between lay and professional bodies of knowledge and can alter the basis of user involvement. Instead of users answering questions or being consulted about recommendations, the users involved in action research can frame the questions and the recommendations. This alters the power relations between researchers, professionals and users and involves the dissemination of health promotion research findings within neighbourhoods and community groups.

Community groups involved in action research are often facilitated or aided by academics or health professionals and may be self-help groups or advocacy groups who have obtained funding for a specific project. A recent example is peer research conducted by Save the Children Fund with adolescent users of mental health services (Laws 1999).

Dissemination through theatre

Rather than text based dissemination through research reports, papers or newspaper coverage, dramatizing research findings for performance to users and professionals is often used. There is a body of work in which theatre is the vehicle used to showcase and disseminate research findings (Mienczakowski 1997). Much of this activity is not evaluated. However, a group in Toronto developed some research-based theatre relating to metastatic breast cancer that was derived from interview transcripts with the advice of two of the interview subjects (Gray *et al.* 2000). The evaluations of the performances by questionnaires both to users and their families and to health professionals indicated that the audiences felt that there was a sense of relevance and that they benefited from seeing it. They felt that 'the fact that the theatre was based on research made it more 'true to life' (Gray *et al.* 2000 p. 140).

Augusto Boal's work on the theatre of the oppressed has been used to encourage the spec-actors to participate in the development of the script and to give voice to marginalized and oppressed groups (Patterson 1994). This approach has recently been used to validate research findings and generate community feedback in a study (the Southern Africa Stroke Prevention Initiative). In addition, puppetry has been used along with street theatre to raise awareness of HIV/AIDS or of domestic violence (Drumbeat@comminit.com).

Barriers to dissemination

There are many barriers to timely and effective dissemination and communication between researchers and users.

Career structures

Academics may only get rewarded for publishing in peer-reviewed journals, rather than providing other forms of dissemination. Professionals may get no time for research or in-service training.

Institutional barriers

Funding may not resource dissemination and it may be difficult for academics, professionals, policy makers and users to meet on neutral ground.

Ownership issues

The funder may assert ownership of the results, or there may be copyright issues, so that the researcher may write the report but be unable to disseminate it to professionals or the community.

Delay of publishing in academic journals

The process of submission, peer review and re-submission can take up to eighteen months. This is often the period during which it would be appropriate to disseminate and yet the results are unpublished.

Technical barriers

The language of research is technical and opaque. Dissemination requires clarity and simplicity of presentation, both visually and verbally, and researchers are not trained in this (Crosswaite and Curtice 1994).

Overcoming barriers to dissemination

It is mistaken to view dissemination as a one-way traffic system of knowledge moving from researchers to implementers. It should be seen as a two-way process between researchers and implementers, and the focus should be on mechanisms and linkages between the two groups (King *et al.* 1998). New knowledge belongs not to the scientists who develop it, but to everyone. Green (1987) argues for more efficient and systematic approaches to research dissemination aimed at the public. Knowledge is often the outcome of problem-solving activities by professionals: this knowledge is then reported by academics, and a closer relationship is needed to 'assume joint responsibility for knowledge creation, development and dissemination' (Eraut 1994 p. 57).

In addition to producing clear briefings on research findings to a variety of audiences using all types of media, it is often apposite to have advisory or steering groups whose membership reflects the constituencies the researchers wish to influence. Ament (1994) proposed six strategies to overcome barriers to dissemination.

1 Publishing in a variety of academic journals and publications that are read by policy makers;

2 Presenting research papers at conferences attended by the policy makers and consumers;

3 Presenting research findings to the groups who took part in studies;

4 Using the mass media to publicize study findings e. g. newspapers, radio, TV;

5 Providing appropriate information to interest groups and lobbyists;

6 Using personal contacts, formal, and informal networks for face-to-face meetings.

There have been several initiatives during the last ten years to narrow the gap between the researchers and the wider community, and the effective dissemination of research findings has become a priority. Funders have recently placed more emphasis on dissemination, and many funding bodies now request that researchers set out their dissemination strategies as part of their funding proposals. There is an increased willingness to fund these activities as part of the research. There is a recognition that dissemination is an integral part of all health promotion research activity and should be built into every programme, from its initial stages through to its completion. It is not an add-on activity.

The Internet

Evaluation of the dissemination of health promotion research on the Internet is a new and important area to cover, in terms of its impact on policy makers, practitioners and service users. The Internet has become an important resource for disseminating research either through electronic journals, or through web pages linked to research centres or charities (Duffy 2000). The openness of access to the Internet means that the distinction as to whether information is for professionals or users has become blurred. The quality of health information is a source of concern and there are journals or journal sections that give guidance on this. For example, the journal *He@lth Information on the Internet* summarizes resources and information on particular subjects as well as publishing articles on experiences in developing information for the web such as the experience of Contact a Family (CaF) in developing a web site (Barnett 2001). One of the ways to evaluate both to whom and to what extent research information on the web is being disseminated is to track the number of 'hits', and get visitors to the site to complete questionnaires so as to provide a profile of users. The use of the Internet has transformed the dissemination of health research findings but access is not available to all, nor is it clear how the information is used.

Evaluating dissemination

Despite the considerable literature emphasizing the importance of dissemination and bemoaning the gap between research and practice, there has been little evaluation of the dissemination of health promotion programmes. What there has been does not have high visibility in the research field (King *et al.* 1998). Nevertheless there are some general issues and examples of good practice. Most of these involve developing linkages to bridge the gap between research and practice, and an evaluation of process as well as outcome.

Examples

A case study evaluating the dissemination of an information resource pack on key research findings and practice implications of a project on women's smoking in the UK showed that two years after the pack was distributed, through professional and organizational networks, it was felt to have been useful to those that had requested it. This

Examples *(Contd.)*

evaluation emphasized the importance of the user-friendly approach in the form of cards, and the importance of using networks for distribution. It showed that if research based findings are presented appropriately for the target audience (in this case professionals) they are likely to use them (Blackburn *et al.* 1997).

The importance of linkage mechanisms and of attention to process is underlined by the failure of the 'Put Prevention into Practice' (PHIP) programme which was developed to address barriers to prevention in family practice. After promoting the kit for two years through the Academy of Family Physicians in the US, only 27% of the members had heard about the programme. The availability of a kit was inadequate on its own and the researchers found a need for linkage mechanisms such as training, continuing medical education, and consultation services (Medder *et al.* 1997).

An example of successful dissemination of a health promotion programme through using linkages is the Canadian Heart Health Initiative, which started as a programme in 1986 with the development of a policy framework and heart health surveys in 10 provinces. Since 1989, all provinces have become involved in heart health demonstration programmes which have been developed through setting up provincial heart health coalitions with between 15–40 community organizations. There were over 40 community interventions ongoing in 1996. Process evaluations of these interventions map 'the extent of community mobilization, leadership development, coalition building, program acceptability and quality' (Stachenko 1996 p. 58).

Dissemination is fundamental to the ethics and practice of applied research in health promotion, and yet both process and outcome evaluations of dissemination are neglected areas. These evaluations must be developed so that effective dissemination can achieve the importance and visibility it deserves. Such evaluation is difficult to fund, but recent developments in health promotion research policy that emphasize the development of evidence-based practice may mean more resources will be available.

Key points

Effective dissemination can be encouraged by:

◆ Enhancing dialogue between researchers and users;

◆ Developing practitioner-based or participatory action research;

◆ Developing dissemination strategies from the beginning of the study;

Evaluation of dissemination requires:

◆ A monitoring of both the process and outcomes using a range of methodologies;

◆ Sufficient resourcing from the initial stages of the project.

References

Almedom, A. M., Blumenthal, U., and Manderson L. (1997) *Hygiene Evaluation Procedures: Approaches and methods for assessing water and sanitation-related hygiene practices.* International Nutrition Foundation for Developing Countries (INFDC),

Ament, L. A. (1994) Strategies for dissemination of policy. *Research, Journal of Nurse-Midwifery,* **39** (5), 329–331.

Barnett, D. (2001) Developing a charity Web Site: the experience of Contact a Family. *He@lth Information on the Internet,* June 4–5.

Blackburn, C., Graham, H., and Scullion, P. (1997) Disseminating research finding on women's smoking to health practitioners: findings from an evaluation study. *Health Education Journal,* **56**, 13–124.

Crosswaite, C. and Curtice, L. (1991) *Dissemination of Research for Health Promotion: A literature review.* Research Unit in Health and Behavioural Change, University of Edinburgh.

Crosswaite, C. and Curtice L. (1994) Disseminating research results – the challenge of bridging the gap between health research and health action. *Health Promotion International,* **9** (4), 289–296.

Duffy, M. (2000) The Internet as a research and dissemination resource. *Health Promotion International,* **15** (4), 349–353.

Entwistle, V. (2000) Developing research-based information: creativity or compromise? *Health Expectations*, **3**, 87–89.

Eraut, M. (1994) *Developing Professional Knowledge and Competence*. Falmer Press, London and Washington.

Glenton, C. and Oxman, A. (1998) The use of evidence by health care user organizations, *Health Expectations*, **1** (1), 14–22.

Gray, R., Sinding, C., Ivonoffski, V., Fitch, M., Hampson A., and Greenberg, M. (2000) The use of research based theatre in a project related to metastatic breast cancer. *Health Expectations*, **3**, 137–144.

Green, L. (1987) Three ways research influences policy and practice: the public's right to know and the scientist's responsibility to educate. *Health Education*, **18**, 44–49.

Green, L. W. and Johnson, J. L. (1996) Dissemination and utilization of health promotion and disease prevention knowledge: theory, research and experience. *Canadian Journal of Public Health*, **87**, (Suppl. 2), 11–17.

Grimshaw, J. M. and Russell, I. T. (1993) Effect of clinical guidelines on medical practice: a systematic review of rigorous evaluations. *Lancet*, **342**, 1317–1322.

Hart, E. and Bond, M. (1995) *Action Research for Health and Social Care*. Open University Press, Buckingham.

King, L., Hawe, P., and Wise, M. (1998) Making dissemination a two-way process. *Health Promotion International*, **13** (3), 237–244.

Laws, S., Armitt, D., Metzendorf, W., Percival, P., and Reisel, J. (1999) *Time to Listen: Young people's experiences of mental health services*. Save the Children, London.

Lewando-Hundt, G., Porter, B., Faerman, M., Lubtzky, H., Goldshtein, E., Waternberg, M., Tessler, H., Rimon, C., Karplus, C., and Galil, A. (1995) Moving towards a family-oriented ethnic sensitive child development service. *Social Sciences in Health*, **1** (1), 45–59.

Medder, J., Sussman, J. L., Gilbert, C., Crabtree, B. F., McIlvain, H. E., McVea, K., Davis, C. M., and Hawver, M. (1997) Dissemination and implementation of put prevention into family practice. *American Journal of Preventive Medicine*, **13** (5), 345–351.

Mienczakowski, J. (1997) Theatre of change. *Research in Drama Education*, **2** (2), 159–172.

Patterson, D. L. (1994) A role to play for the theatre of the oppressed. *The Drama Review*, **38** (3), 37–49.

Potvin, L. (1996) Methodological challenges in evaluation of dissemination programs. *Canadian Journal of Public Health*, **87** (Suppl. 2), 279–283.

Richardson, A., Jackson, C., and Sykes, W. (1990) *Taking Research Seriously: Means of improving and assessing the use and dissemination of research*. HMSO, London.

Rogers, E. M. (1983) *Diffusion of Innovations*. The Free Press, New York.

Stachenko, S. (1996) 'The Canadian Health Health Initiative: Dissemination perspectives. *Canadian Journal of Public Health*, **87** (Suppl. 2), S57–59.

Chapter 13

Conclusions
Integrating methods for practice

Margaret Thorogood and
Yolande Coombes

Health promotion has come of age. No longer the poor cousin of
public health, it has taken its place as a key component of public
health strategy, and that is amply demonstrated in this book. The
examples used range from preventing malaria in children in Malawi,
to smoking cessation in Scotland; from intimate partner violence to
routine clinical screening.

Health promotion grew out of two movements. There was an
increasing awareness that the reactive treatment of people who seek
help from health professionals would never have a major impact on
the health of populations. At the same time there was a growing
mutual interest of both researchers and practitioners from many disciplines in developing new ways of thinking about health and ill
health. In health promotion, ill health is seen not merely as a collection of diseases for which biomedicine seeks cures, but as a limitation
to taking control of one's life – which is why health promoters refer to
'health as a resource for everyday living' (see Chapter 1). In health
promotion, the biomedical and quantitative disciplines, using mecha-
nistic models of health, meet and merge with the qualitative social
sciences, where health is viewed holistically, as an expression of the
relationship between an individual and the society in which he or she
lives. It is small wonder that health promotion has been described as a
'Multidisciplinary Tower of Babel' (Kelleher 1998).

We did not intend that this book would comprise a complete
enumeration of all the languages in the Tower, that is, all the available

methods for evaluating health promotion. Indeed, we doubt that any definitive list of such methods could be drawn up, since new approaches are constantly being developed. However, we have aimed to discuss some of the most topical and important issues that have bearing on the development and refinement of health promotion evaluation. Health and health promotion are multifaceted constructs; they need multidisciplinary perspectives and methods to be understood. For health promotion to achieve the effects that are intended, it is important that the holders of these various perspectives work together rather than in isolation. Different disciplines are mutually interdependent in the evaluation of health promotion.

In this book we have brought together some of those disciplines, showing how the different disciplinary perspectives provide a multi-dimensional, richer and more informative portrait of an intervention. In addition we have tried to include discussion of some of the problems that can arise as researchers climb over disciplinary walls, and meet in what is still a sketchily mapped, new disciplinary area. The process of evaluation is contributing to the professionalization of health promotion and this, in itself, is a consequence of the emergence of evaluation as an acknowledged way of validating knowledge. Some disciplines, such as physics, have clear laws (although never unchangeable) based on scientific experiment; other disciplines, such as anthropology, involve the validation of knowledge through discussion and debate from opposing epistemologies. In the evaluation of health promotion the whole range of disciplinary approaches have a valid place.

We have aimed to include a wide spectrum of examples from diverse cultural and economic contexts. In the last few years there has been a movement, energetically led by the World Health Organization, to engage seriously and on a worldwide scale with those health problems that account for the greatest burden of ill health. As a consequence, the concepts, behaviour models, and techniques of health promotion have been rolled out in many new, and often very poorly resourced, contexts. This movement presents new challenges for health promotion, and we have aimed to reflect some of these new challenges in this book. However, Berridge's historical perspective (Chapter 2) provides an important reminder that new concepts of health promotion and of evidence-based practice are culturally defined, and sit within an historic tradition which can be traced back to the activities of Edwin Chadwick, who sought to reduce the burden of poverty by improving the health of the poor. Some of the most recent writers on health promotion have turned Chadwick's reasoning on its head, arguing that a reduction in the burden of ill health can only be achieved by improving the economic conditions of the poorest people in society. Berridge also reminds us that the concept of evaluation itself is historically contingent on social processes.

Several authors in this book have noted the importance of planning evaluation alongside the planning of the programme that is to be evaluated. Evaluation should become part of an intervention from the start, and the design of the evaluation should be an integral part of the initial design. Evaluations that are bolted on to already functioning interventions are rarely satisfactory, almost always lacking baseline data, and often lacking clarity about the original or evolved aims of the project.

When an intervention is first being designed, the objectives should be explicitly stated and agreed by all stakeholders. The objectives of an intervention are the key criteria against which any evaluation must measure the outcome. This means that a prerequisite of designing an evaluation is a definition of the objectives of the intervention. These are often not explicitly stated, and there can sometimes be profound disagreements between different stakeholders. Wellings and Macdowall (Chapter 11) write about the circular process of evaluation, where the results of evaluation act as formative feed back into the evolving design of the intervention. Seeking defined, relevant and realistically achievable objectives of a health promotion initiative can sometimes be a powerful formative evaluation in itself. By contrast to Wellings and Macdowall's discussion of the circular nature of evaluation (the feedback loop), Platt *et al.* (Chapter 6) describe a situation where it became important *not* to feedback the results of a process evaluation during the course of the project. They also discuss some of the other complexities involved in carrying out process evaluation, not least the need to accommodate diversity and constantly adjust to changes during the implementation of the project.

The same prerequisite of defining objectives at the start applies to the evaluation itself. As Coombes (Chapter 3) and Chapman (Chapter 7) both argue, the first stage of evaluation should involve a consideration of what the evaluation is needed for, and what actions will be taken as a result of the evaluation report. It is increasingly the case that every initiative that is funded is required to be evaluated. The danger, then, is that the evaluation itself will compromise the effectiveness of the intervention. It is a mistake to set up complex and expensive evaluation programmes, requiring detailed data that would not otherwise be collected, without first considering what those data will be used for. The monetary and human resources provided for the evaluation should be proportionate both to the resources used in the health promotion initiative and to the use that is to be made of the evaluation report. Evaluations do not need to be complex, expensive and focused on distal outcomes in order to be useful. In many situations, simple process evaluations of proximal outcomes are all that is needed (Chapter 3). However, as Stevens demonstrates, an important aspect of evaluation must focus on the resource implications of a strategy. Whatever the economic circumstances, resources are always finite and one aim of evaluation should be to ensure that resources are used to maximal effect.

It is also important that evaluation is as objective as can be achieved. For this reason it is important to separate the evaluator from the evaluated. Often those that are carrying out an intervention also carry out the evaluation, but as Wellings and Macdowall (Chapter 11) suggest, that this can mean that the evaluation lacks objectivity.

Defining the relevant recipients of health promotion is sometimes a problem. For example, as Jewkes points out (Chapter 9), most of our interventions are aimed at the community, but we are not always clear who belongs to the community. Jewkes poses the question: is it possible for us to define the community? Britton and Thorogood (Chapter 5) show how the 'gold standard' of evaluation, the randomized controlled trial, has a contribution to make to the evaluation of health promotion, but caution us of some of the pitfalls in adapting this method to the complex world of health promotion. Marks (Chapter 10) reminds us that the ethics of obtaining informed consent is as relevant in health promotion interventions as it is in a clinical trial of a new drug, while Lewando-Hundt and Al Zaroo (Chapter 12) remind us that the people that we research or intervene with are joint owners of the results or new knowledge, and that dissemination is therefore an ethical obligation.

As health promotion develops into a mature discipline, it is apparent from this book that it will need a combination of approaches to evaluations using a variety of methods to shed light on the vast arena in which health and health promotion take place. Neither qualitative nor quantitative approaches should be considered easier or, conversely, more rigorous than the other. What is essential is that methods are used appropriately for the job in hand, and are used to evaluate those areas of health promotion activity where they are most able to increase our knowledge and evidence base. No one approach should be considered the exclusive domain of one group of researchers. Within the health promotion Tower of Babel we must learn each other's disciplinary language, and learn respect for each other's culture, because only then can the best, most informative evaluations be carried out.

Key points

- Evaluation should be designed at the same time that the intervention is planned, and adequate resources should be allocated.
- Effective evaluation of health promotion interventions and programmes requries a multi-method approach. No one method or theory is adequate.
- The evaluation should be designed according to the purpose for which it is required.
- The rights of the participants in health promotion must be considered.

References

Kelleher, C. 1998 Evaluating health promotion in four key settings. In J. K. Davies and G. MacDonald *Health Promotion Striving for Certainties*. Routledge, London.

Index